I0803750

IMAGES
of America

GUTHRIE
100 YEARS OF HEALTH CARE

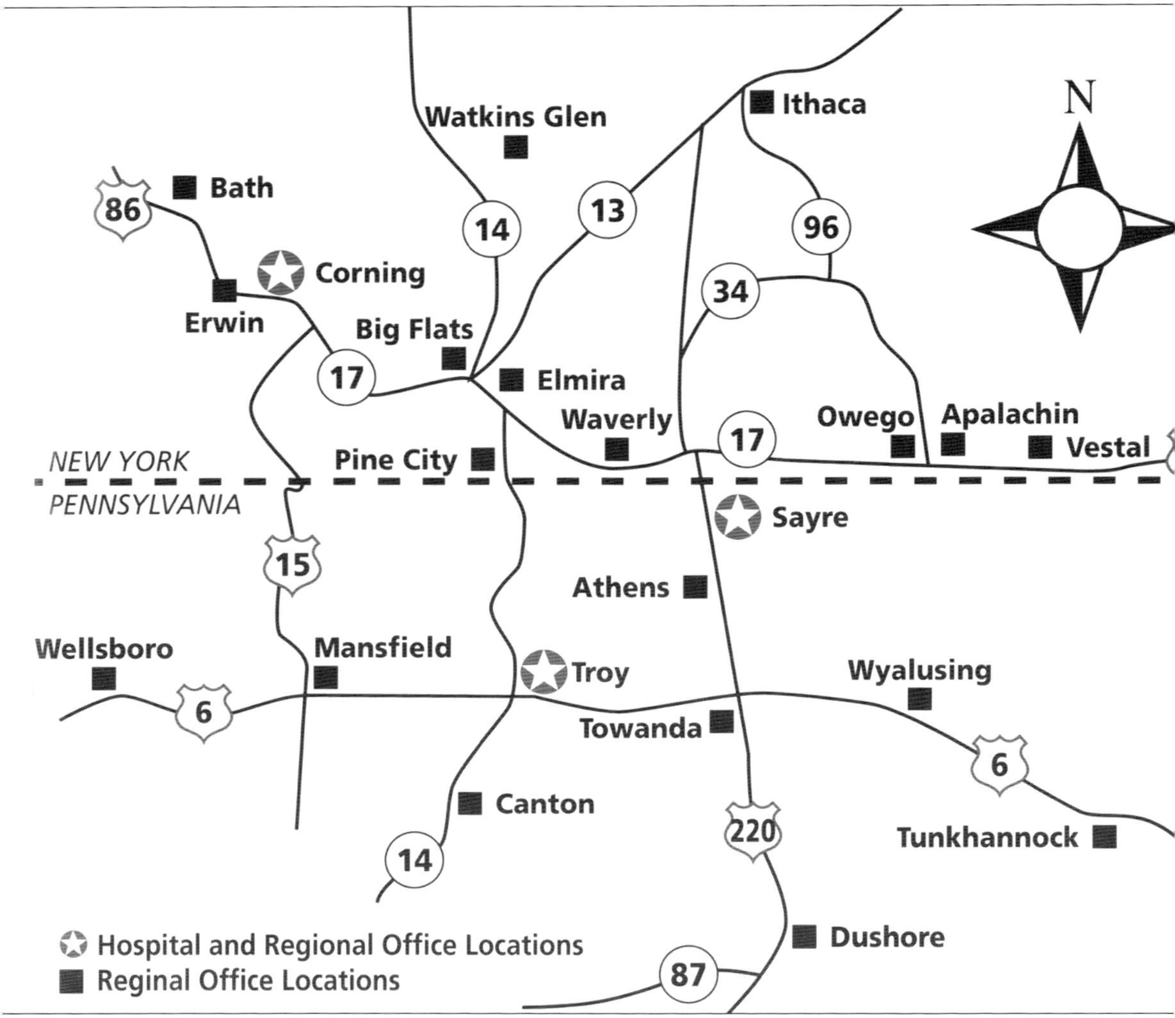

This map shows the locations of Guthrie Clinic physician offices and Guthrie Healthcare System hospitals and facilities in 2009—nearly 100 years after Dr. Donald Guthrie brought his vision for a multi-specialty group practice to Sayre. From a small country hospital to an integrated health care delivery system, Dr. Guthrie's values continue to be the foundation on which the organization stands. The health care system now includes more than 360 physicians and providers and 4,000 employees. (Courtesy of the Guthrie Archives.)

ON THE COVER: Dr. E. Star Judd (left), surgeon at the Mayo Clinic, performs an operation with Dr. Donald Guthrie during Dr. Guthrie's surgical training. This photograph was taken at the Mayo Clinic in Rochester, Minnesota. (Courtesy of the Guthrie Archives.)

IMAGES
of America

GUTHRIE
100 YEARS OF HEALTH CARE

Guthrie Archives

ARCADIA
PUBLISHING

ISBN 978-0-7385-7221-5

Published by Arcadia Publishing
Charleston, South Carolina

Printed in the United States of America

Library of Congress Control Number: 2009930759

For all general information contact Arcadia Publishing at:
Telephone 843-853-2070
Fax 843-853-0044
E-mail sales@arcadiapublishing.com
For customer service and orders:
Toll-Free 1-888-313-2665

Visit us on the Internet at www.arcadiapublishing.com

This pictorial history serves as a record of the legacy of Dr. Donald Guthrie and is dedicated to all the physicians and staff who served with him, as well as those who came after.

Contents

ACKNOWLEDGMENTS

This brief look back in time at the Guthrie era would not have been possible without the support of the leaders of Guthrie Health: Dr. Joseph A. Scopelliti, president and chief executive officer, Guthrie Clinic, and co-chief executive officer, medical affairs, Guthrie Health; and Mark Stensager, president and chief executive officer of Guthrie Healthcare System and co-chief executive officer, administrative affairs, Guthrie Health.

The Guthrie Archives collection, unless otherwise noted, is the source of information and pictures included in this publication. This book would not have been possible without the use of some of the many hundreds of images stored in the archives. The dedication of the volunteers, employees, physicians, and others who carefully saved documents and photographs or researched, sorted, and cataloged all manner of Guthrie artifacts and memorabilia for the archives over the years is much appreciated.

The authors would also like to thank corporate communications staff members Brian Denlinger, graphic designer, and Wendy Hankle, public relations associate, who devoted many hours to scanning these images and editing the text.

INTRODUCTION

Today it is hard to imagine what life was like in 1910 in rural America. Most small towns had no paved roads, homes were lit with gaslights, people traveled on foot or via horse-drawn carriages, and it often took days to get to the next town.

At the beginning of the 20th century, Sayre was home to the bustling Lehigh Valley Railroad rail yard. More than 70 acres of buildings, or shops, were used to build or repair train engines and railcars. Employing several thousand men, the rail yard was a sea of activity as work was done on top of and underneath these large and heavy iron machines. The work was dangerous, injuries were common, and the medical care provided through the dispensary was quite primitive.

Judge Asa Packer owned the Lehigh Valley Railroad. He was an entrepreneur who had interests in many businesses, including railroads, coal mining, and water navigation systems. His son, Robert Asa Packer, took over as president of the railroad after his father's death and moved to Sayre. He built a lavishly appointed mansion on a small rise overseeing the shops. Following Robert Asa Packer's death, community leaders approached his sister, Mary Packer Cummings, who had inherited the mansion, to ask if they might use it for a hospital. She agreed, asking that the hospital be named after her brother.

Although better equipped than the rail yard dispensary, in those days people were somewhat distrustful of hospitals, and most medical and nursing care—even surgery—was provided at home. At first the hospital grew slowly, and its initial patients were rail yard workers who paid one day's salary in return for one year of hospital care, should they need it. By the beginning of the 20th century, the hospital and its staff had gained the acceptance and confidence of the community, and the hospital was starting to make a name for itself for excellent patient care. In addition to rail yard workers, townspeople and others from around the area were now using its services.

Into this setting came a well-trained and ambitious young surgeon. Dr. Donald Guthrie, fresh from a three-year surgical internship at Mayo Clinic in Rochester, Minnesota, could have undoubtedly started his career anywhere he chose. His family lived in Wilkes-Barre, and his father was also a physician. However, Dr. Guthrie was so influenced by the way in which medicine was practiced in the rural setting of Mayo Clinic that he chose to come to Sayre.

Dr. Guthrie believed that people living in the country had as much right to excellent medical care as those living in large cities. His vision was to create a multi-specialty group practice of physicians whose expertise in many areas of medicine and surgery could be focused on providing the best treatments possible. Under Dr. Guthrie's leadership, Robert Packer Hospital and the clinic that bore his name became synonymous with high-quality care.

Just a few years after coming to Sayre, Dr. Guthrie started to add specialists to his staff, and by 1920, he brought 11 physicians to Sayre. In 1928, the four-story Guthrie Clinic building opened with 27 physicians. Fundamental to Dr. Guthrie's approach to providing excellent patient care was his belief that education and research were as important to patients' outcomes as bedside care. Just as he received training under the watchful eyes of Drs. William and Charles H. Mayo, so too did two successive generations of Mayo surgeons who were sent to Robert Packer Hospital to train under Dr. Guthrie.

In addition to welcoming interns to train under him and his staff, Dr. Guthrie was very supportive of the hospital's nurses and school of nursing. He led a successful community drive to build a new nurses' residence, which opened in 1926. This was only the first of many building projects undertaken during Dr. Guthrie's tenure. His dedication to his patients' welfare, skills as a surgeon, and personal drive and charisma made him a very successful advocate of the hospital and its needs for nearly five decades.

The railroad, the industry that spawned Sayre, the need for a hospital, and the growth of Guthrie Clinic also served as an import~~ant life~~line decades after Dr. Guthrie's arrival. Many of the patients who came from a distance came by rail, as roads around Sayre were often unpaved or impassable in the winter. Dr. Guthrie had his own railcar, which he used often as he traveled up to 100 miles to provide consultations for other physicians in the region or to give lectures in the major cities of the East Coast.

Dr. Guthrie's arrival in rural Sayre may have seemed inauspicious at the time, but his vision, energy, and unwavering devotion to advancing the care of patients led to the creation of a medical center unrivaled in the region. His reputation as a surgeon and as an exacting chief of staff brought patients from far and wide to the clinic and hospital.

His time at the helm resulted in several expansions of the medical facilities. Following a fire in 1933 that destroyed a major portion of the hospital, he quickly raised the funds to build a bigger and better building. Dr. Guthrie also managed to keep the hospital running during the Great Depression and two world wars, each of which had a significant impact on American life.

An unassuming man of short stature—he often stood on a box to perform surgery—Dr. Guthrie did not let anything derail his dream to bring the best possible medical care to this rural region of the country. His death in 1958 left a void in the clinic and hospital. But, true to the ideals upon which he started his practice, those who worked with him picked up the baton he had passed to them.

Dr. Guthrie was a force unto himself, a larger-than-life man of great intelligence and compassion whose personal and professional philosophies became the foundation on which Guthrie Clinic stands today. His belief in teamwork, excellence, and patient-centered care are the values that guide all of Guthrie Health 100 years after he came to a little rural town in northeast Pennsylvania to follow his dream.

One

Dr. Donald and Emily Baker Guthrie

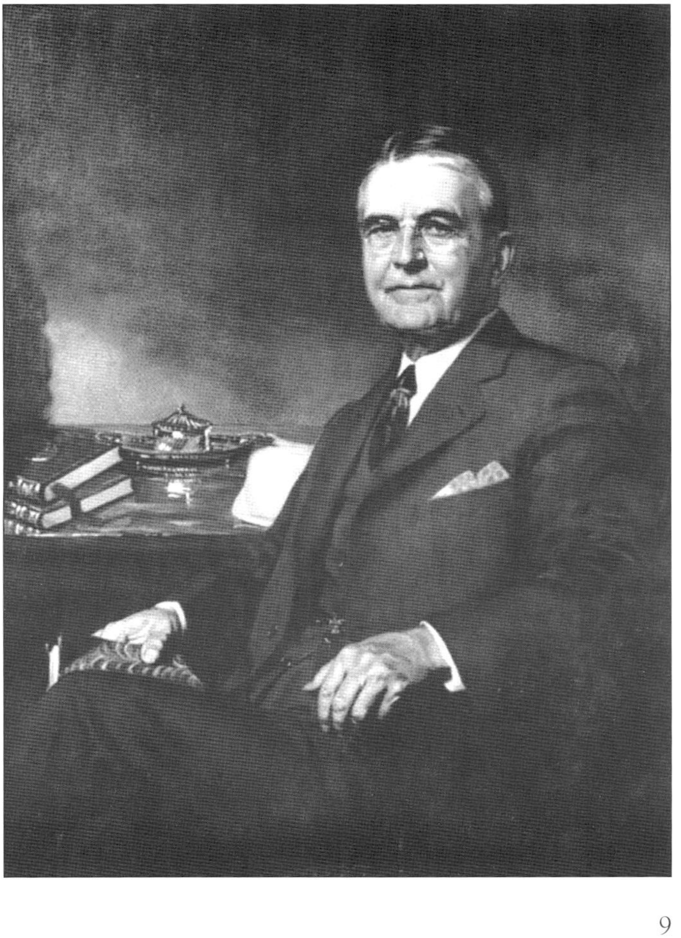

Dr. Donald Guthrie was the founder of Guthrie Clinic and chief of staff at Robert Packer Hospital in Sayre from January 10, 1910, to October 30, 1958. During Dr. Guthrie's 48 years at the helm, he led the transformation of a small country hospital into a major medical center and clinic.

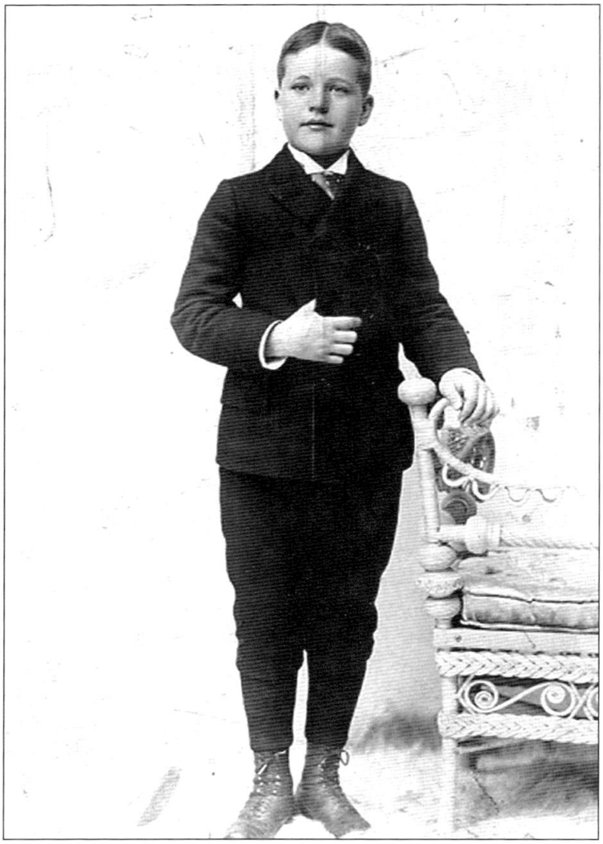

Dr. Donald Guthrie was born on June 23, 1880, to Dr. George and Sarah Hollenback Guthrie of Wilkes-Barre. Dr. Guthrie traced his genealogy to Matthias Hollenback, a pioneer settler of Athens, Pennsylvania.

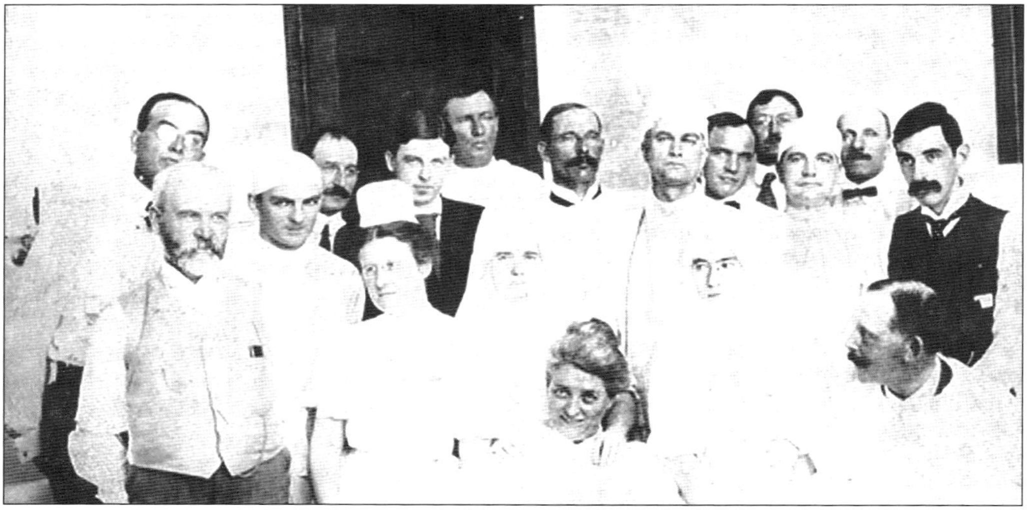

Dr. Guthrie spent three years and four months as an intern at Mayo Clinic in Rochester, Minnesota, where he assisted in nearly 4,000 operations. In this photograph taken at Mayo Clinic, Dr. Guthrie is third from the right. Beside him, also in surgical attire, is Dr. William Mayo; Dr. E. Star Judd is third from the left. Others in the photograph are Dr. Augustus W. Stirchfield, Florence Henderson, Sister Joseph, Sister Sylvester, and Sir Harold Stiles.

This picture of Dr. Guthrie was taken around the time he came to Sayre in 1910.

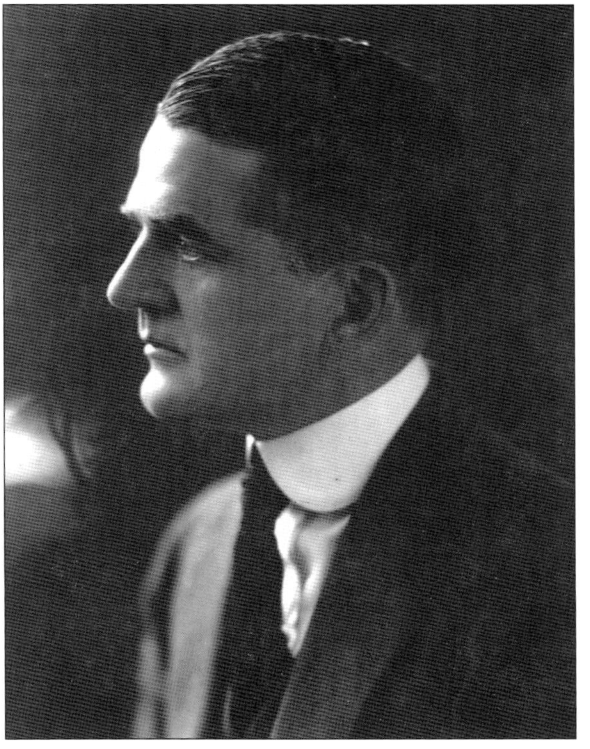

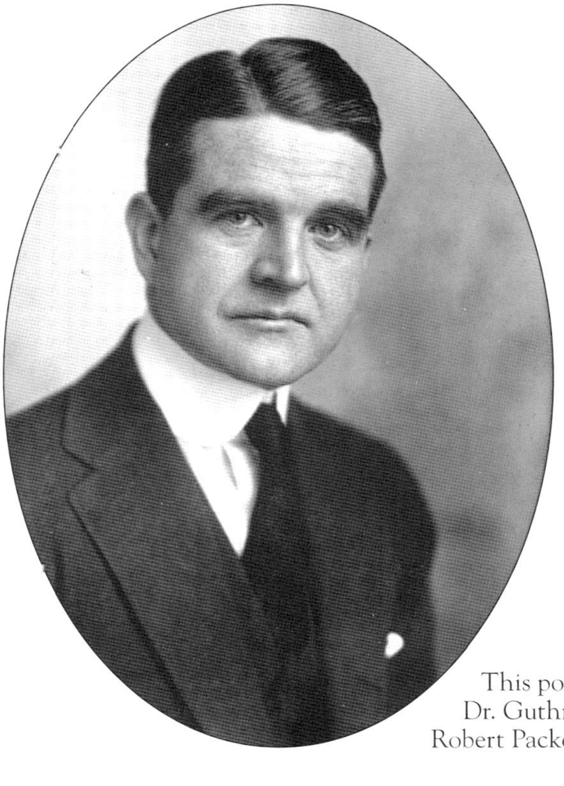

This portrait was taken in 1920 on the occasion of Dr. Guthrie's 10th anniversary as surgeon in chief of Robert Packer Hospital.

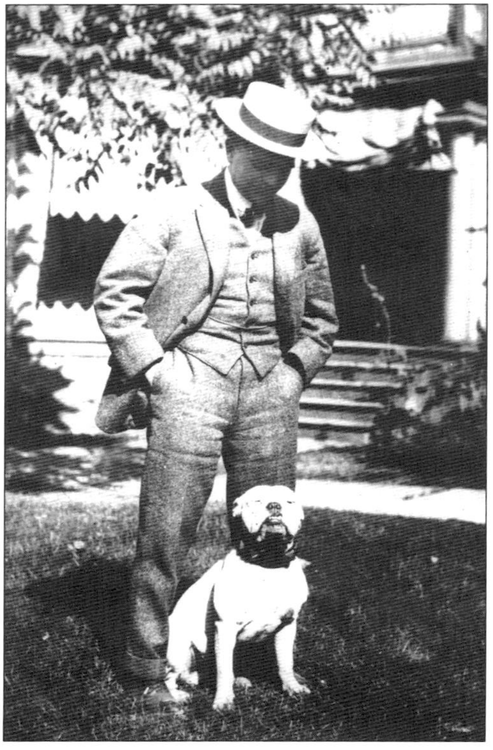

Dr. Donald Guthrie enjoyed the company of his dog Rip Van Winkle.

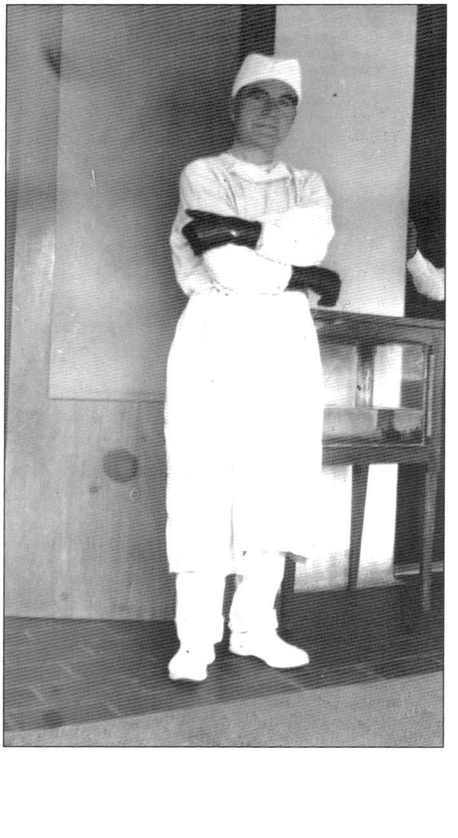

Titled "The Perfect Friend," this photograph shows Dr. Guthrie in surgical attire.

Dr. Guthrie served as program chairman at an event honoring the management and employees of the Athens plant of Ingersoll Rand Company on August 24, 1942.

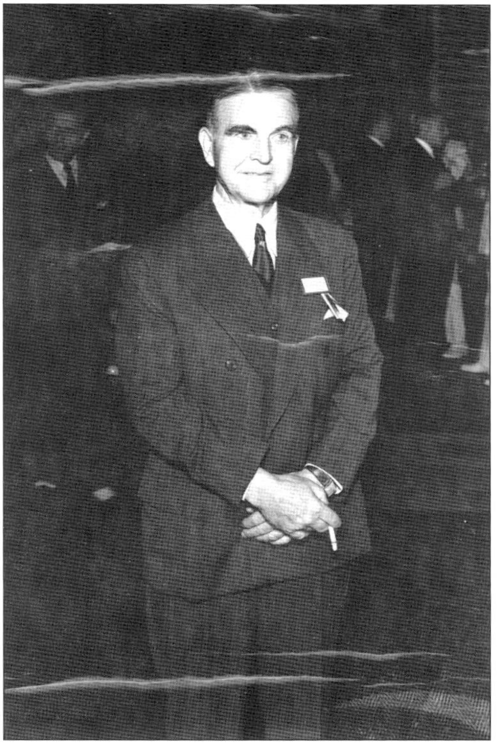

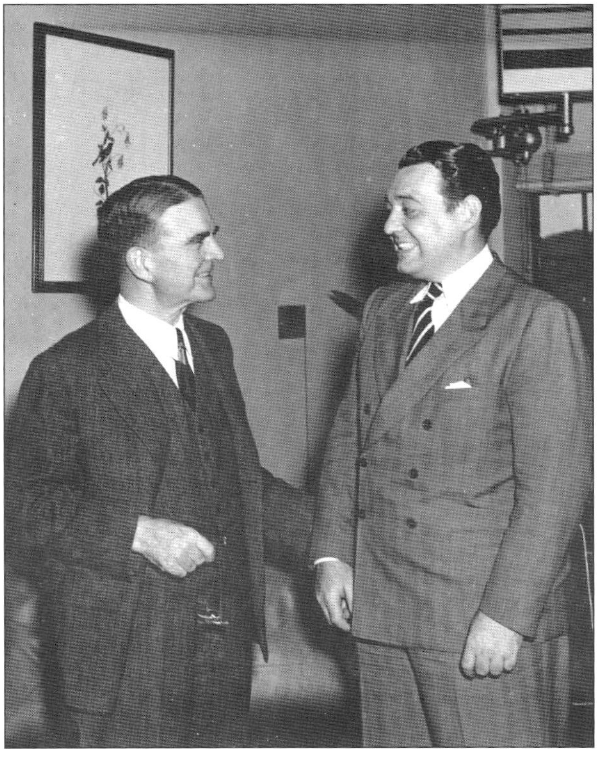

Dr. Guthrie (left) greets businessman Samuel F. Pryor, who served on the board during Dr. Guthrie's tenure. Pryor played an indispensable role in the development of Pan American Airways during the airline's glory years of 1925–1945.

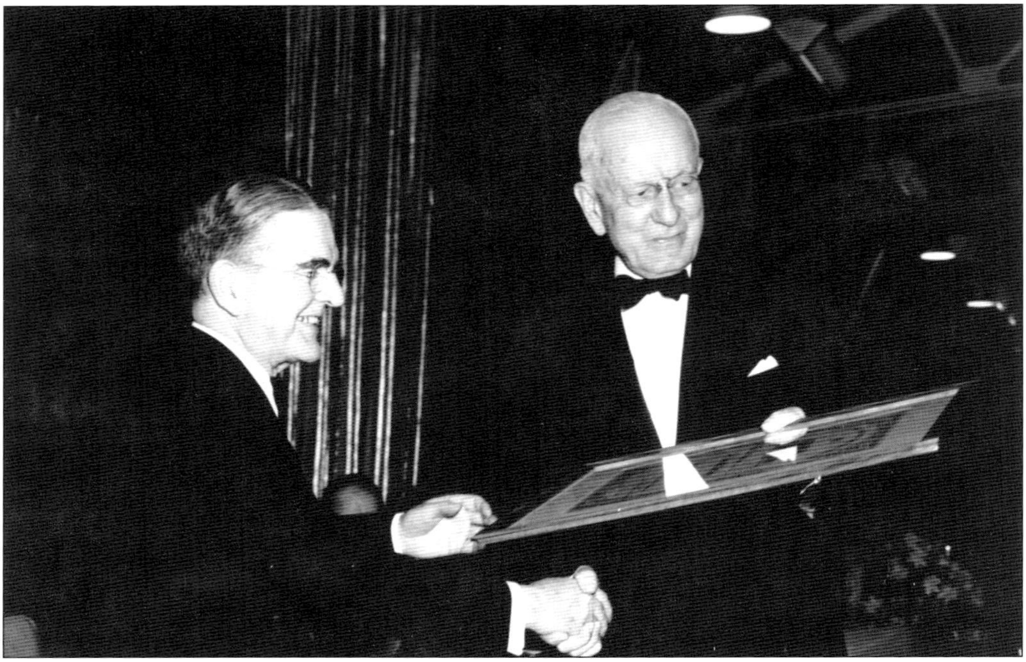

Dr. Donald Guthrie (left) and Thomas Watson, founder of International Business Machines (IBM), share the stage at a celebration. As president of IBM, Watson oversaw the growth of the company into an international force.

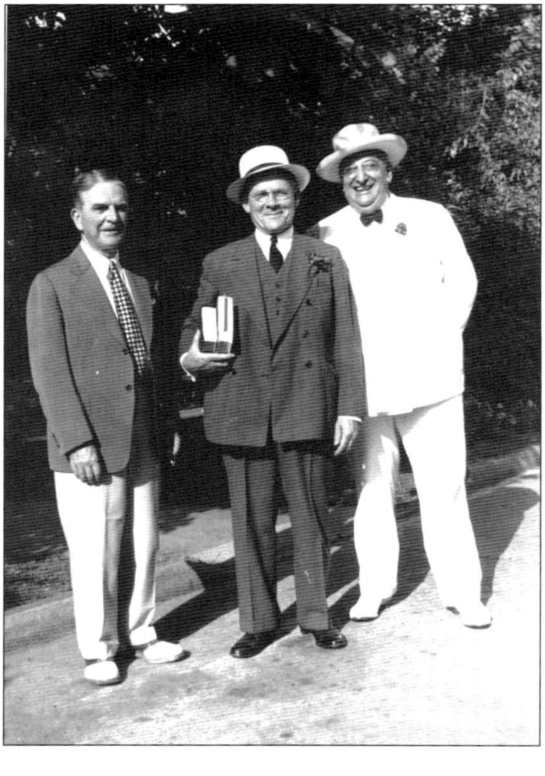

Dr. Guthrie (left) stands next to Arthur James (center), governor of Pennsylvania from 1939 to 1943. The gentleman at right is unidentified.

Near the end of his career as a surgeon, Dr. Guthrie is pictured here in his surgical gown and cap.

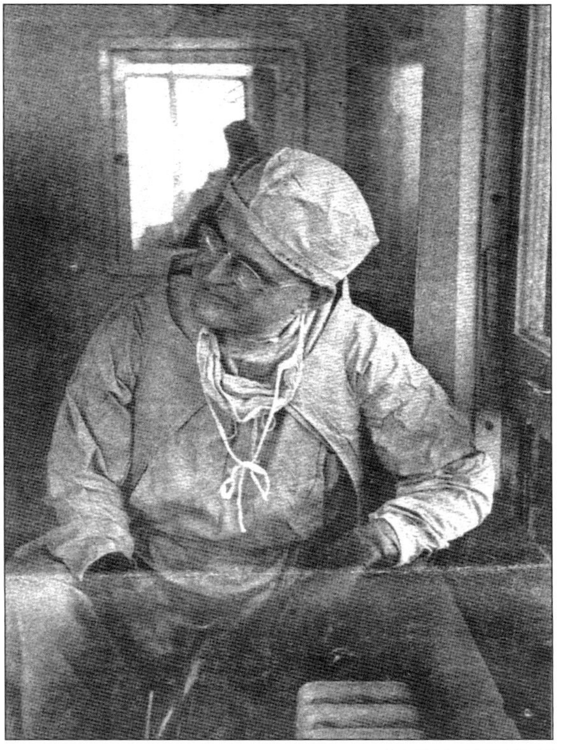

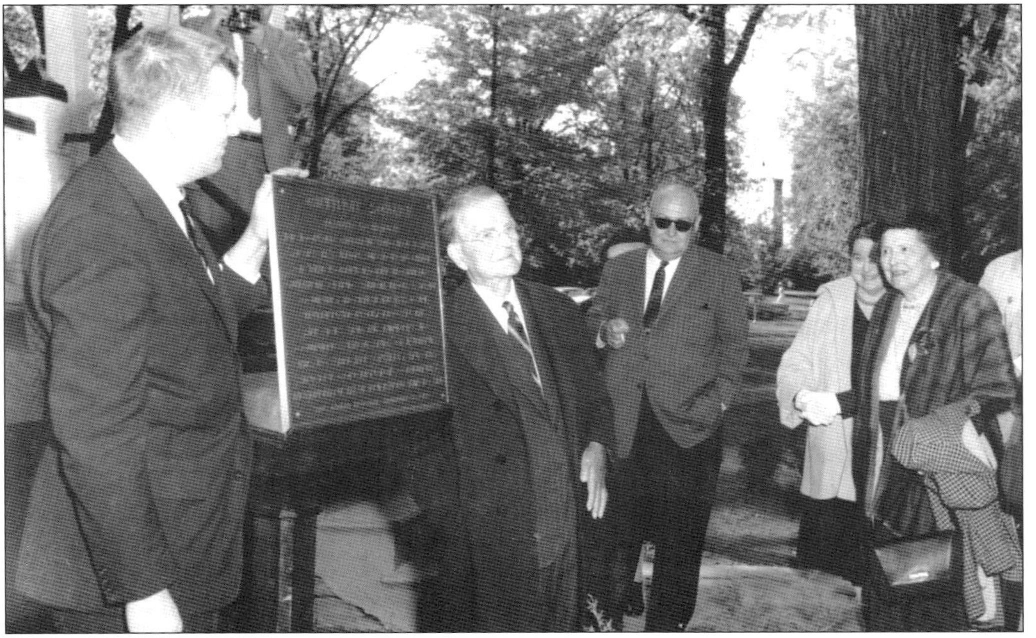

A ceremony dedicating Guthrie Square was held on September 28, 1957. Dr. Guthrie's devotion to the community was honored with a plaque later mounted on a large granite boulder. Guthrie Square is located in Howard Elmer Park in Sayre, across the street from Robert Packer Hospital and Guthrie Clinic. In failing health at the time, this was his last public appearance.

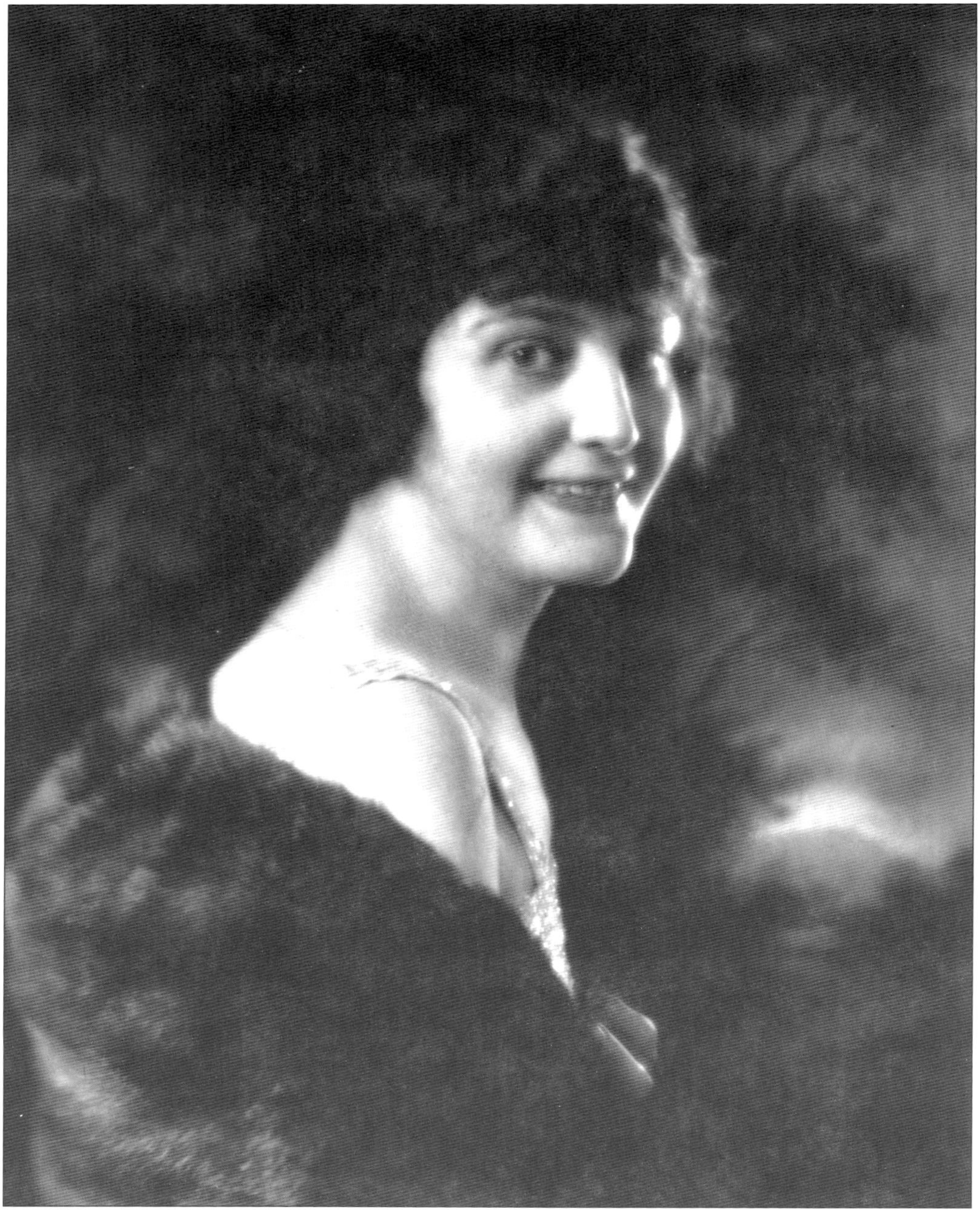

Emily Baker Guthrie married Dr. Donald Guthrie in New York City on December 2, 1916. Known as "Gerry" to her friends, she was born in Brooklyn to Thomas and Emma Baker. Her uncle, Herbert Baker, was vice chairman of Socony-Vacuum Oil Company and a generous donor to Dr. Guthrie's enterprises over the years. When she died in 1976 at 85, the residue of her estate, totaling more than $16 million, was left to Robert Packer Hospital and the Donald Guthrie Foundation for Medical Research.

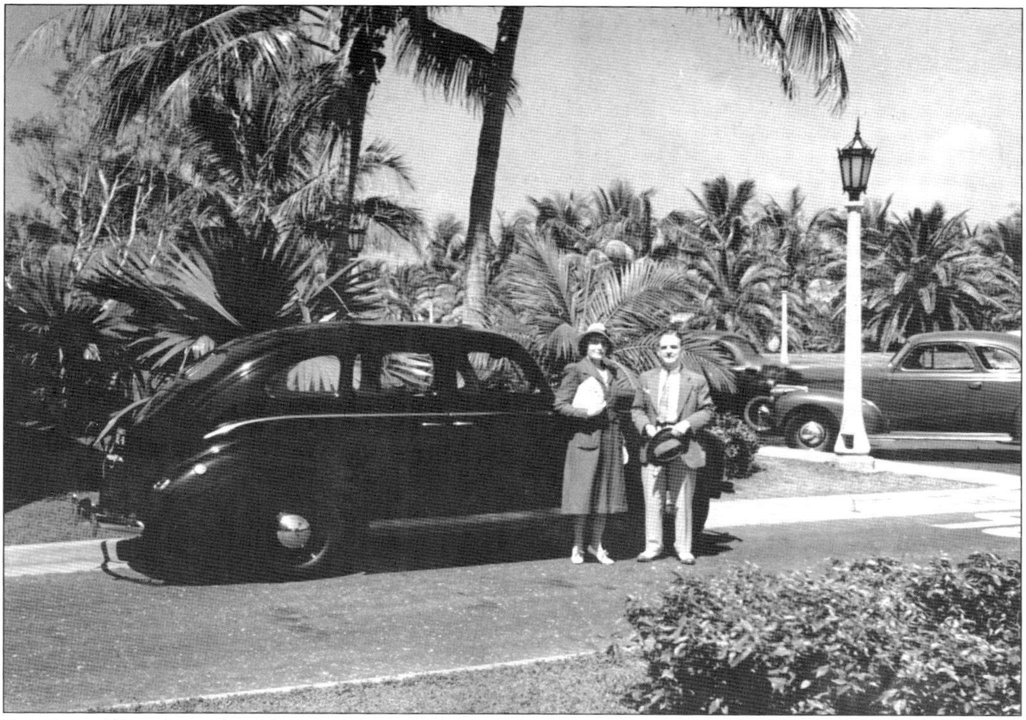

Dr. Donald and Emily Baker Guthrie are shown here on a trip to Florida.

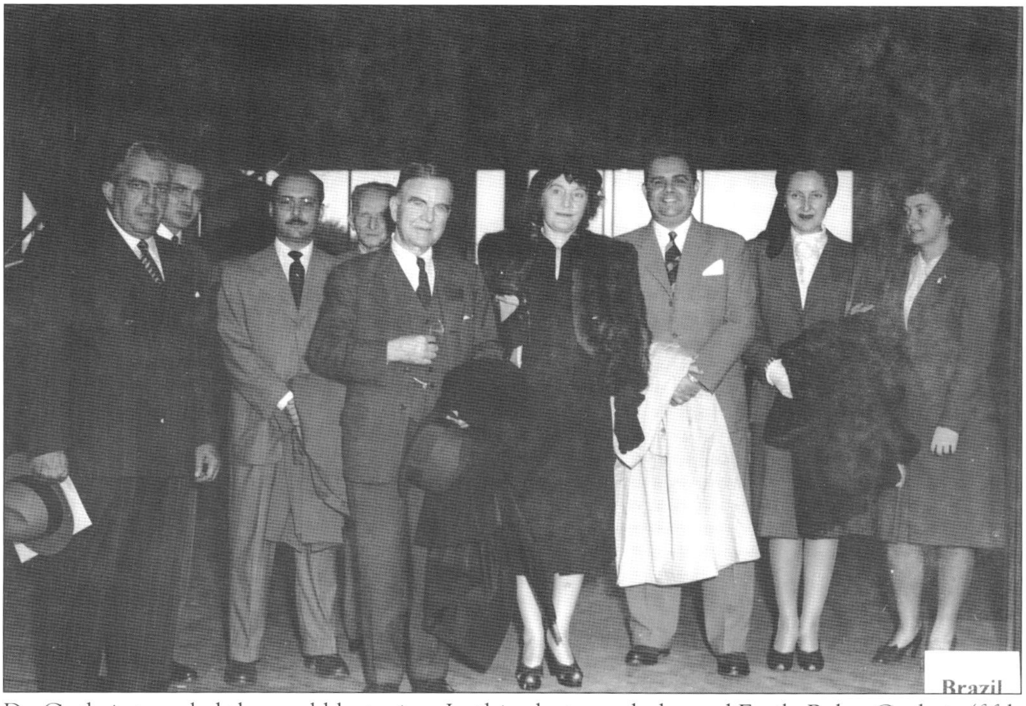

Dr. Guthrie traveled the world lecturing. In this photograph, he and Emily Baker Guthrie (fifth and sixth from the left) are in Brazil.

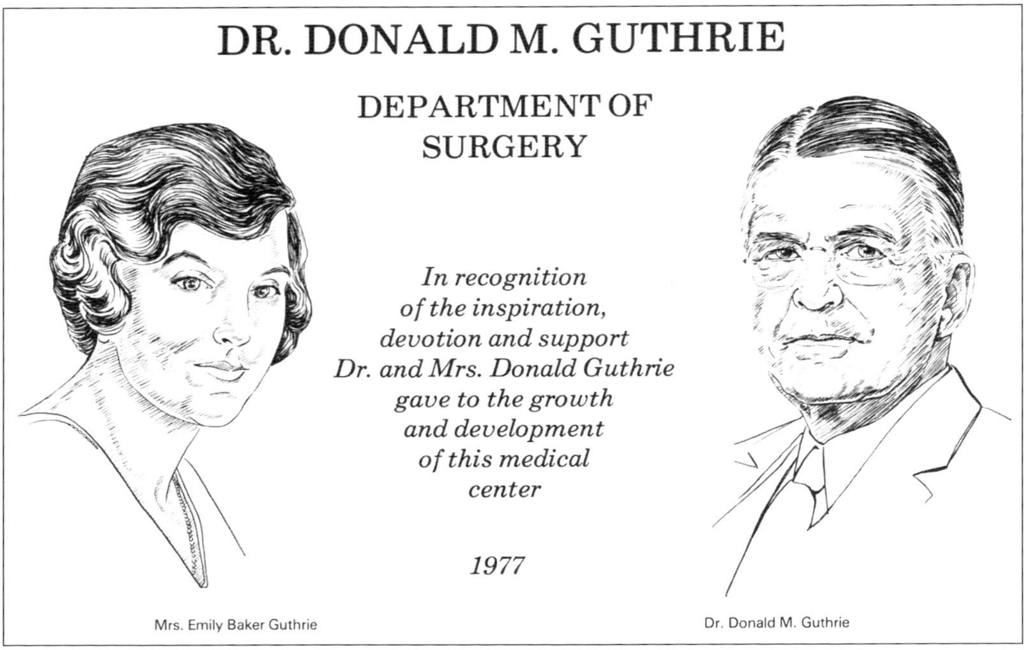

The surgical suite at Robert Packer Hospital, completed in 1977, was dedicated to Dr. Donald and Emily Baker Guthrie.

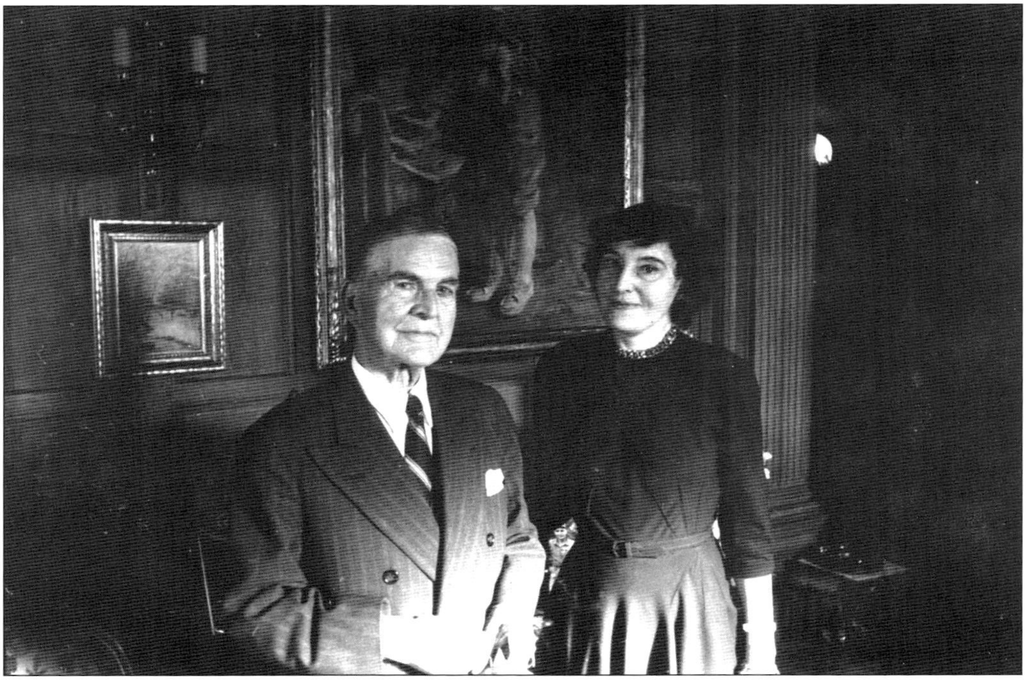

Dr. Donald and Emily Baker Guthrie resided in the chief surgeon's house on the Sayre campus of Robert Packer Hospital and the clinic.

Two

SAYRE AND THE LEHIGH VALLEY RAILROAD

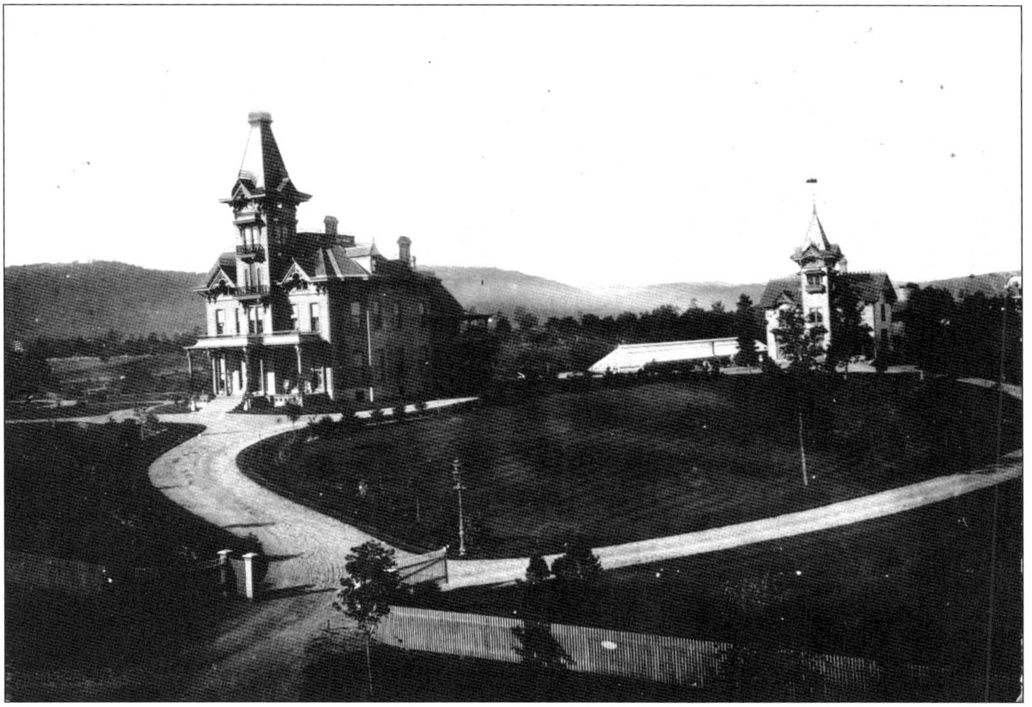

Robert Packer Hospital was named after Robert Asa Packer, who came to Sayre when the town became the point of distribution for the Lehigh Valley Railroad's northern traffic. Shortly after his arrival, Packer invested in the Sayre Land Company and purchased 20 acres between Lockhart and Hayden Streets and between Wilbur Avenue and what was known as Hayden's Pond. On the latter piece of property, he erected Packer Mansion, shown in this photograph (left). The mansion was completed in 1877 and later became Robert Packer Hospital.

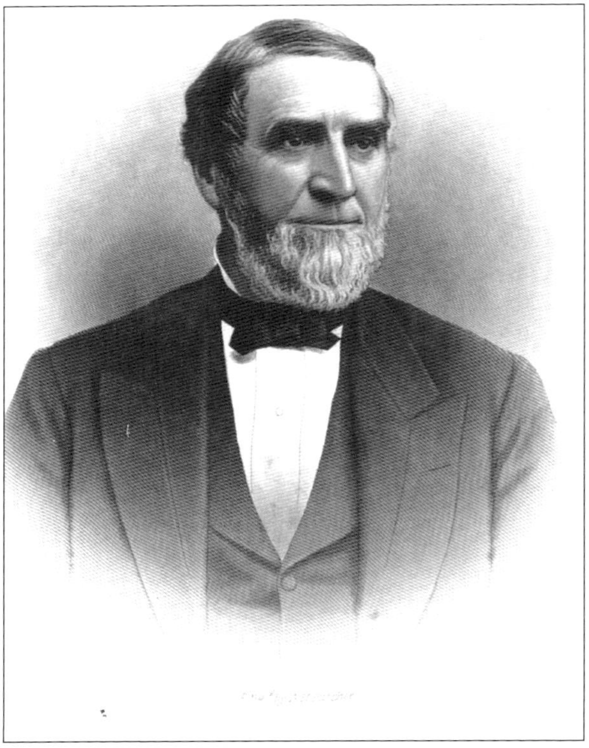

Robert Asa Packer's father, Judge Asa Packer, developed the Lehigh Valley Railroad with the intention of connecting it to the Erie Railroad to facilitate the transport of coal from northern Pennsylvania to the growing cities of the West. Sixty acres of land were purchased in Athens Township and eventually became the Borough of Sayre.

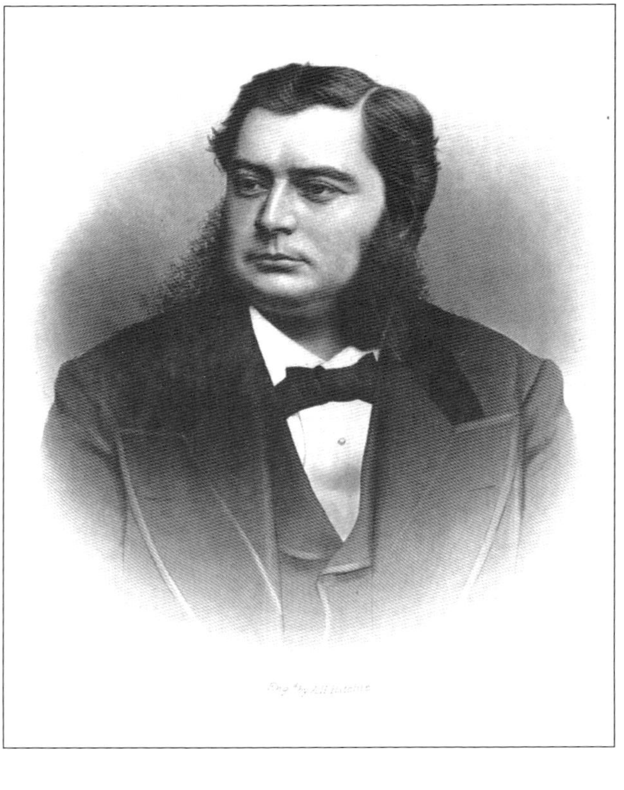

Known as "Bob" to his friends, Robert Asa Packer was born in Mauch Chunk (now Jim Thorpe) on November 19, 1842. After attending Polytechnic Institute in Troy, New York, he joined the Lehigh Valley Railroad as chief of the corps of engineers. He was later president of the Pennsylvania and New York Railroad, as well as the Geneva and Ithaca and Athens Railroads. It was said that Packer was a man of more-than-ordinary business ability, "quick to see the merits of any question and prompt to decide." Packer died on February 20, 1883, in Jacksonville, Florida, at age 40.

Emily Victorine Piollet Packer, daughter of Col. Victor Piollet of Wysox, married Robert Asa Packer in early September 1875. After her husband's death, she married Robert Eggleston, cashier of Lincoln National Bank of New York City. When Packer Mansion was given to the community of Sayre for a hospital, she became a staunch supporter of the organization.

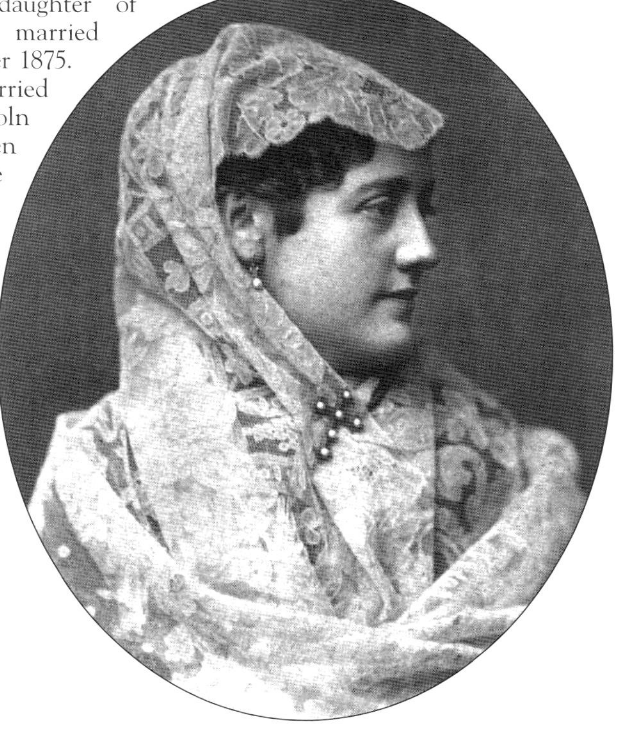

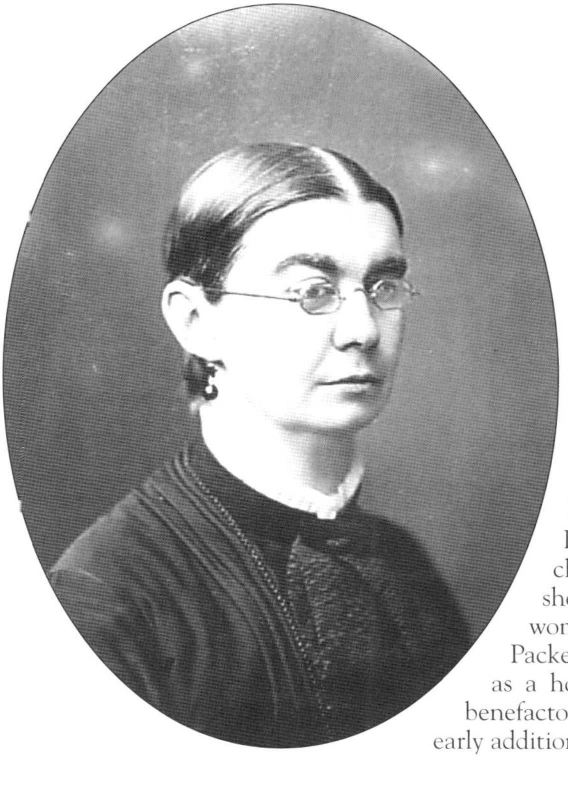

Mary Packer Cummings, sister of Robert Asa Packer, was the last surviving child of Judge Asa Packer. At one time, she was said to be the second-wealthiest woman in the world. Cummings donated Packer Mansion to the people of Sayre for use as a hospital in 1885, and she was a generous benefactor, giving the money needed for most of the early additions and renovations.

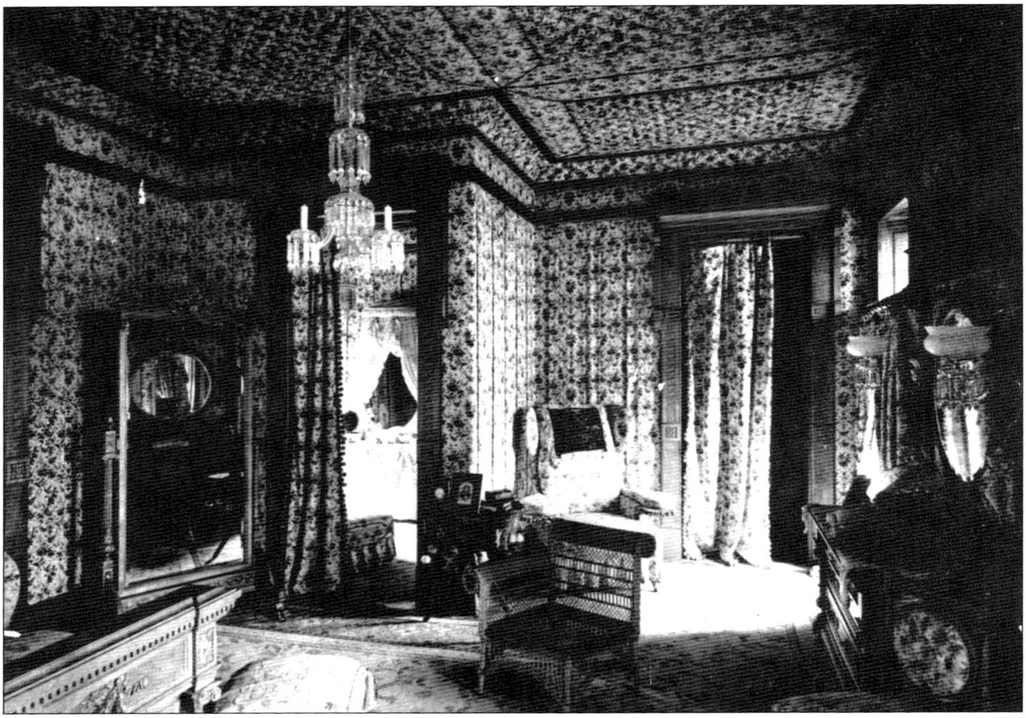

Packer Mansion contained several bedrooms. This one, photographed in 1877, was decorated in true Victorian style.

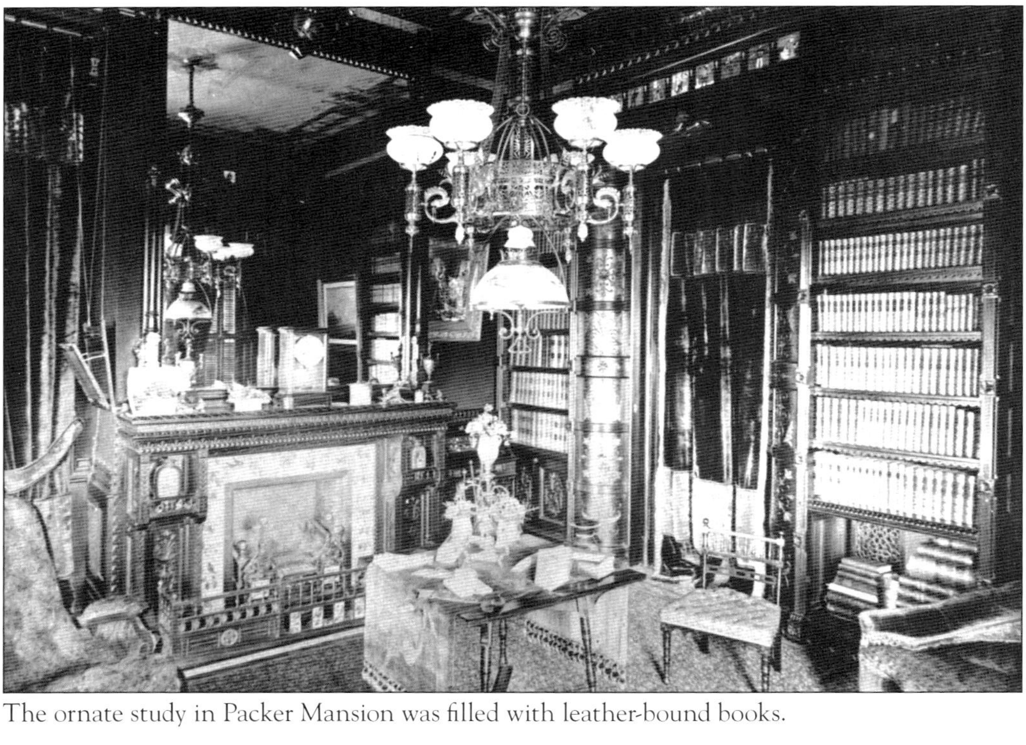

The ornate study in Packer Mansion was filled with leather-bound books.

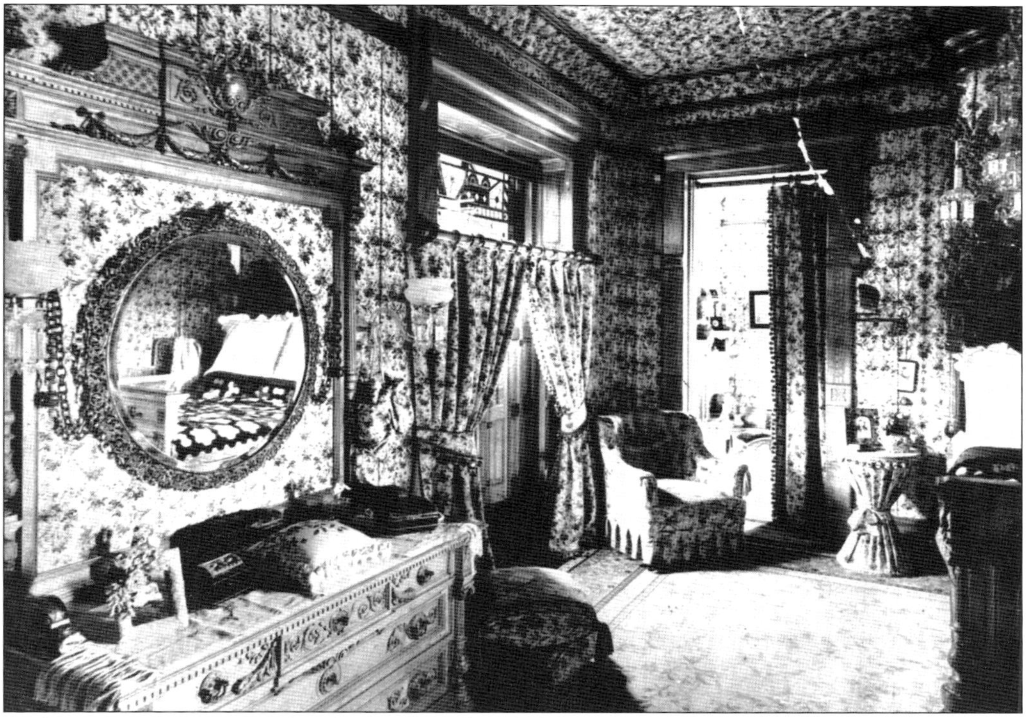

Packer Mansion was completed in 1877 and included this grand bedroom.

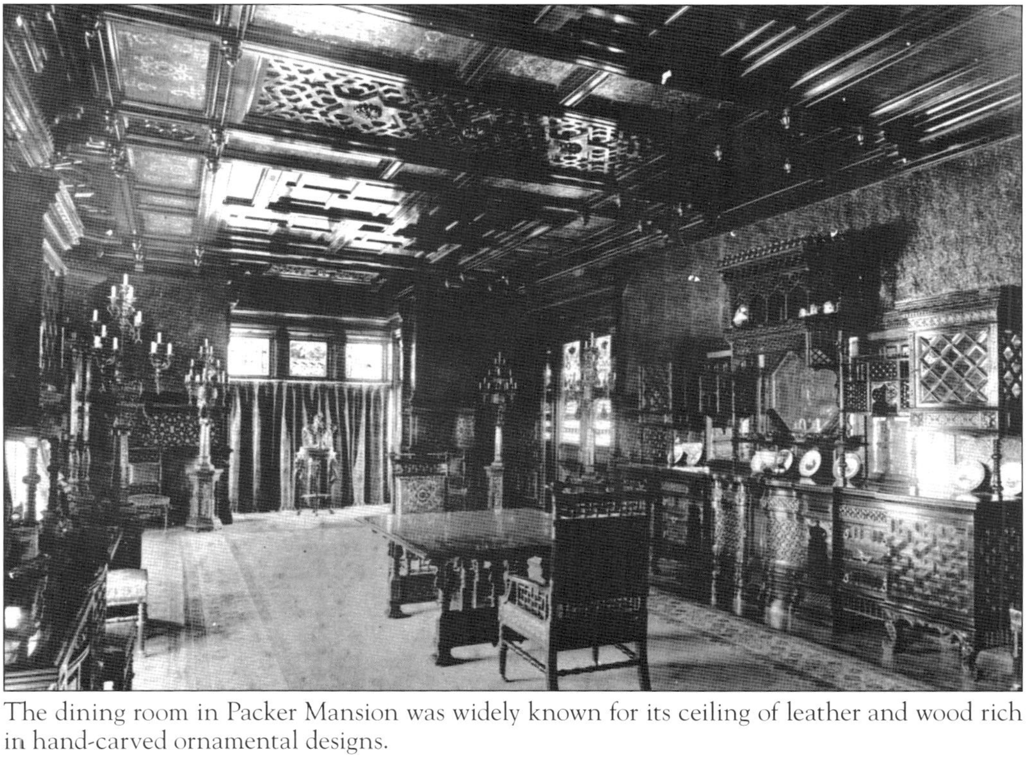

The dining room in Packer Mansion was widely known for its ceiling of leather and wood rich in hand-carved ornamental designs.

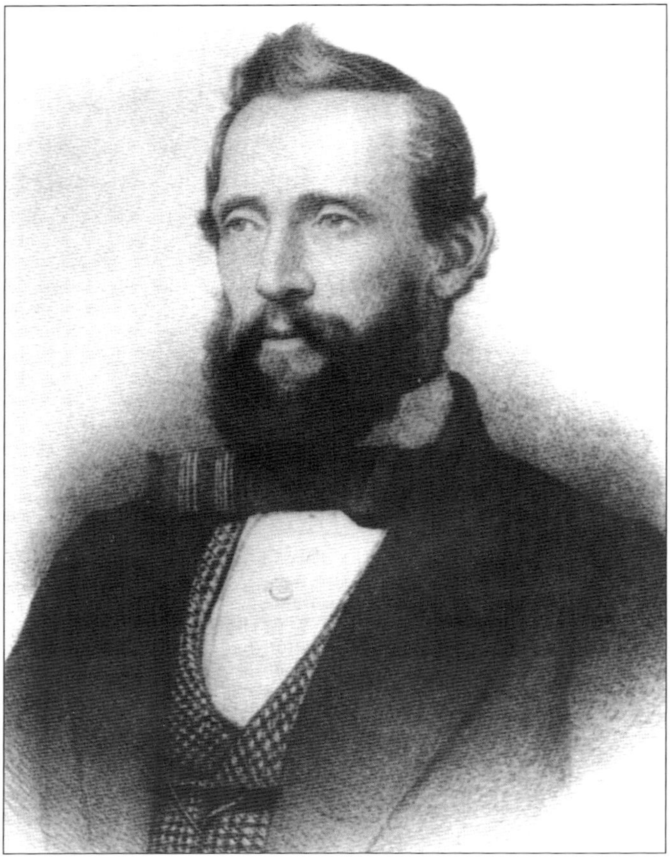

Robert H. Sayre was the chief engineer for the construction of the Lehigh Valley Railroad. As the railroad pushed through northern Pennsylvania, the line came to the junction of the Southern Central Railroad and the Ithaca and Athens Railroad at a station between Waverly and Athens. Howard Elmer founded the Borough of Sayre by renaming the junction and acreage around it in honor of the Lehigh Valley Railroad's chief engineer.

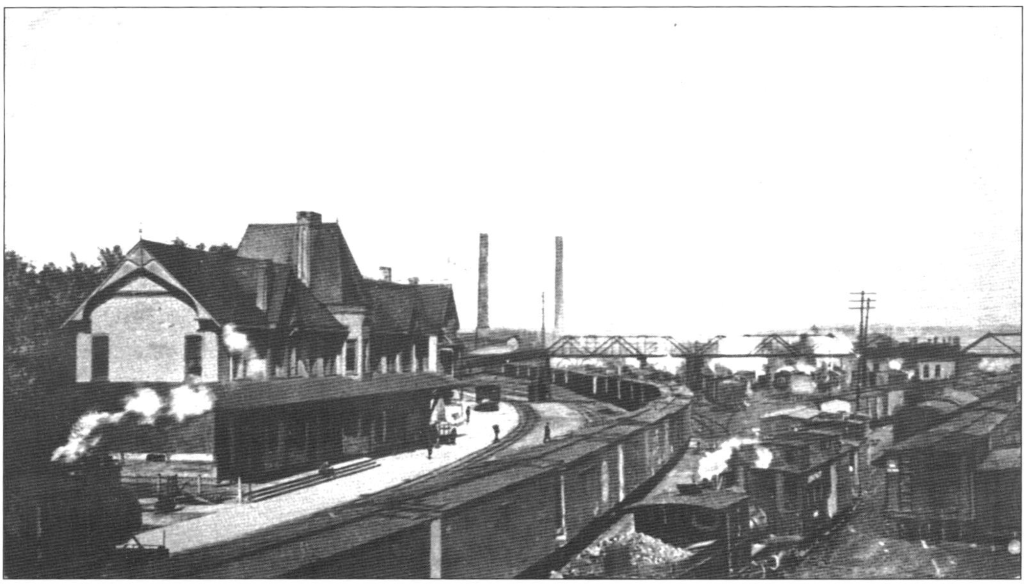

The Lehigh Valley Railroad was a hub of activity in the late 1800s, apparent in this photograph of the crowded rail yards in Sayre.

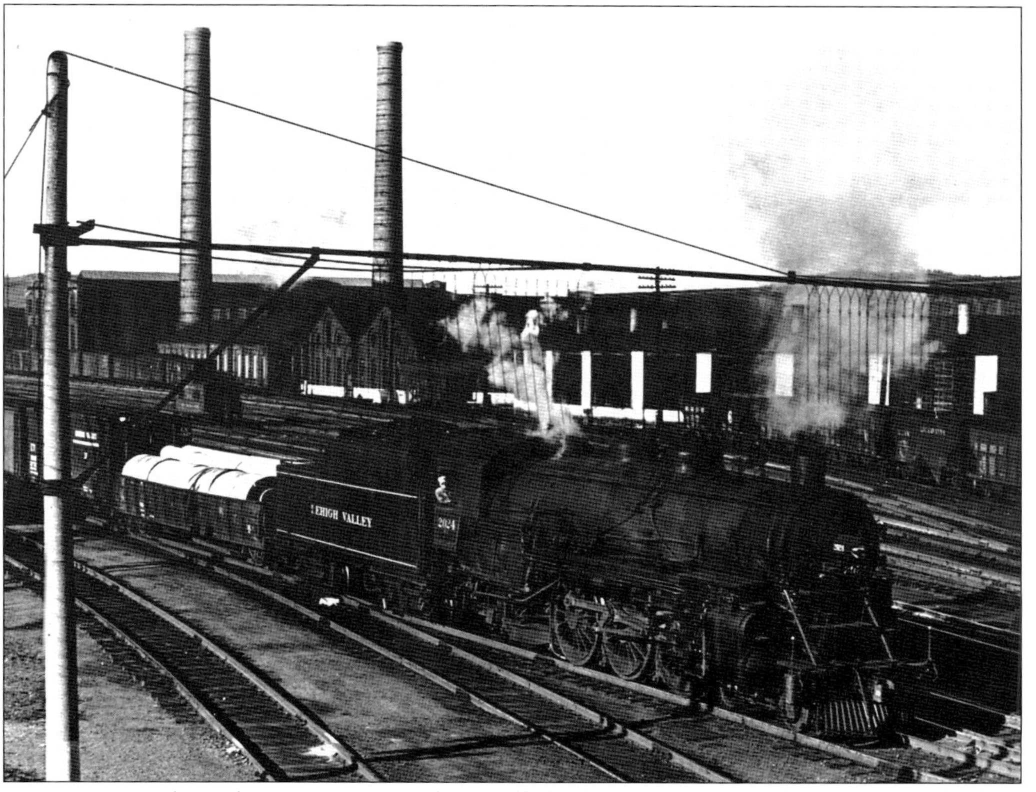

Vast in size and number at one time, almost all the buildings in this photograph of the "big shops" of the Lehigh Valley Railroad rail yard are gone today.

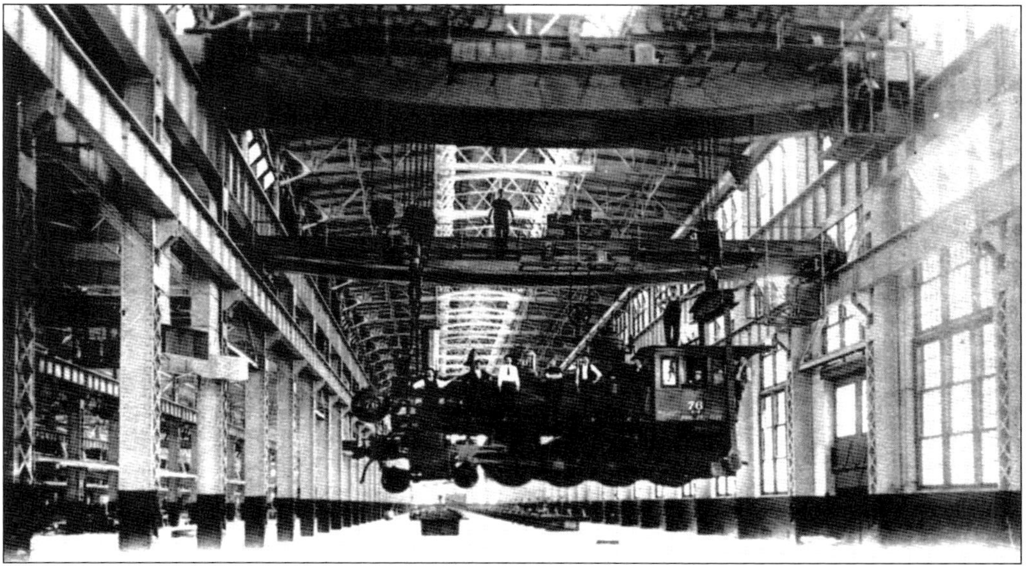

Inside the Lehigh Valley Railroad big shops in Sayre, engines are hoisted for repair.

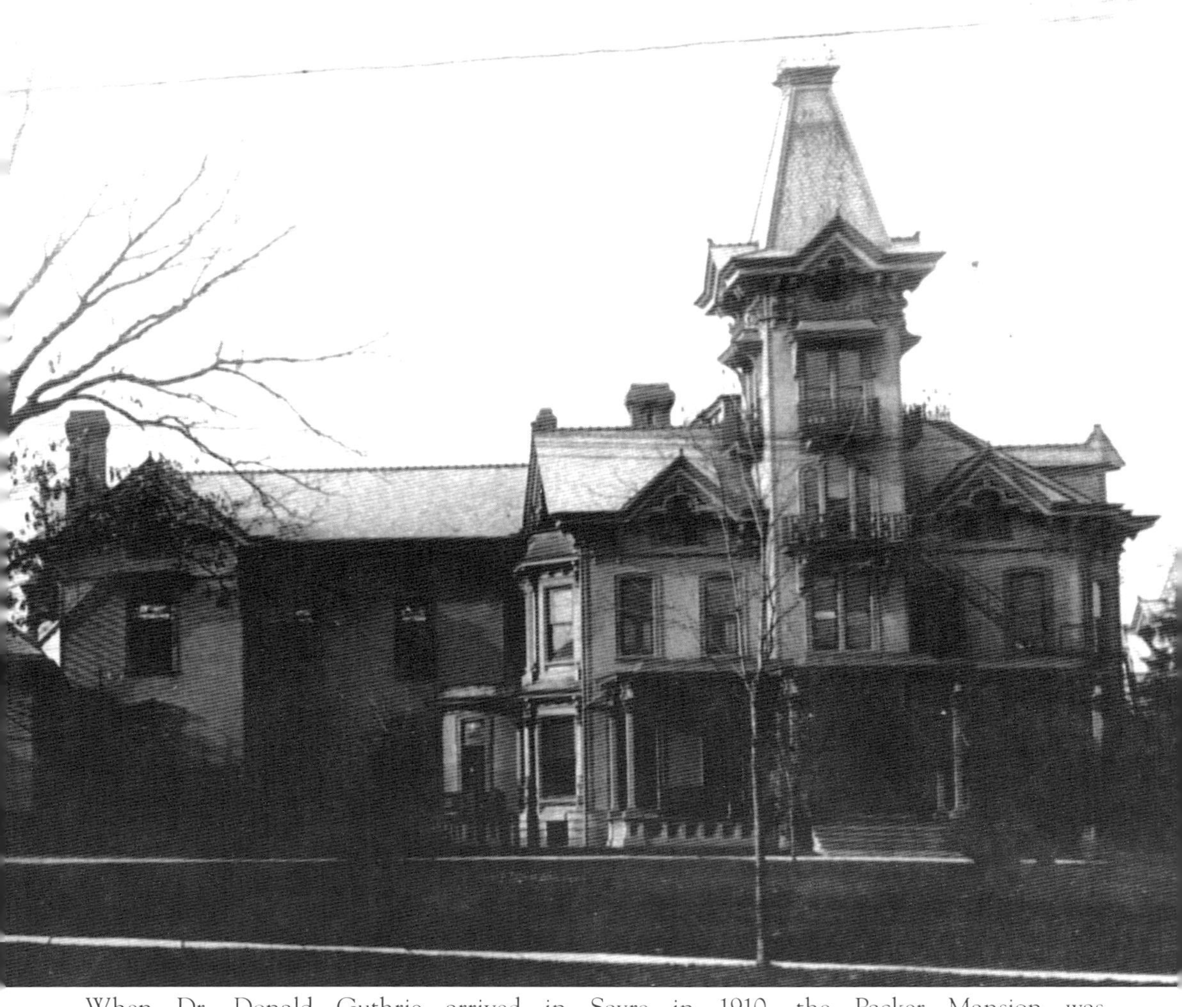

When Dr. Donald Guthrie arrived in Sayre in 1910, the Packer Mansion was an impressive presence.

Three

THE GUTHRIE ERA BEGINS

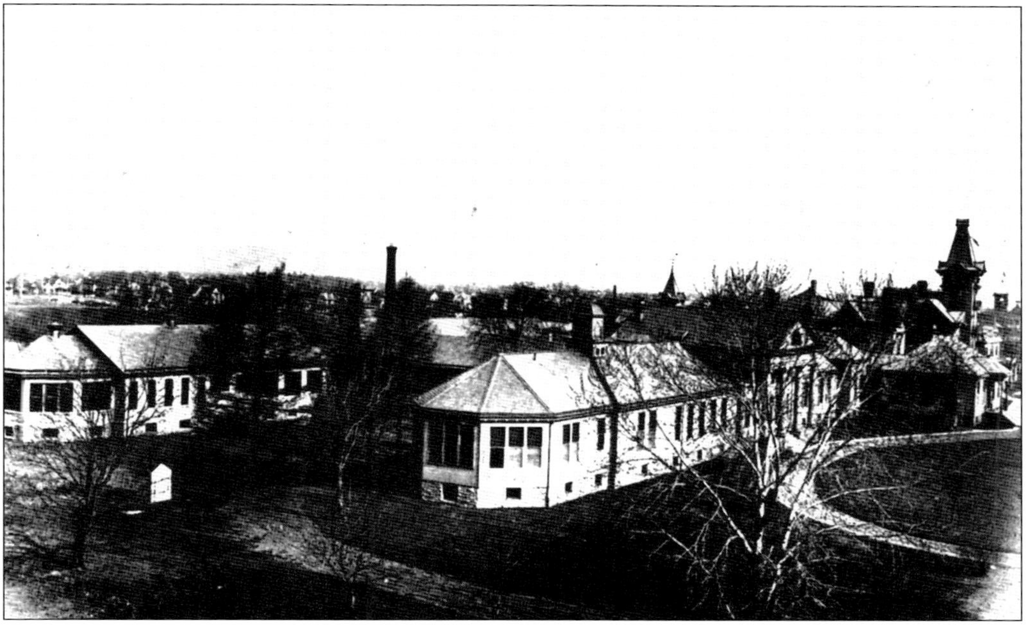

In 1914, Robert Packer Hospital had grown tremendously from the original space of the former Packer Mansion (spire visible on the right) due to Dr. Donald Guthrie's arrival in 1910. As hospital superintendent and chief surgeon, Dr. Guthrie began increasing the size of the medical staff, the size of the facility, and the number of patients treated at the hospital. On February 1, 1912, the eye, ear, nose, and throat department was established. In 1913, the pathological department was added, followed by the urological and medical departments. The Guthrie era had truly begun.

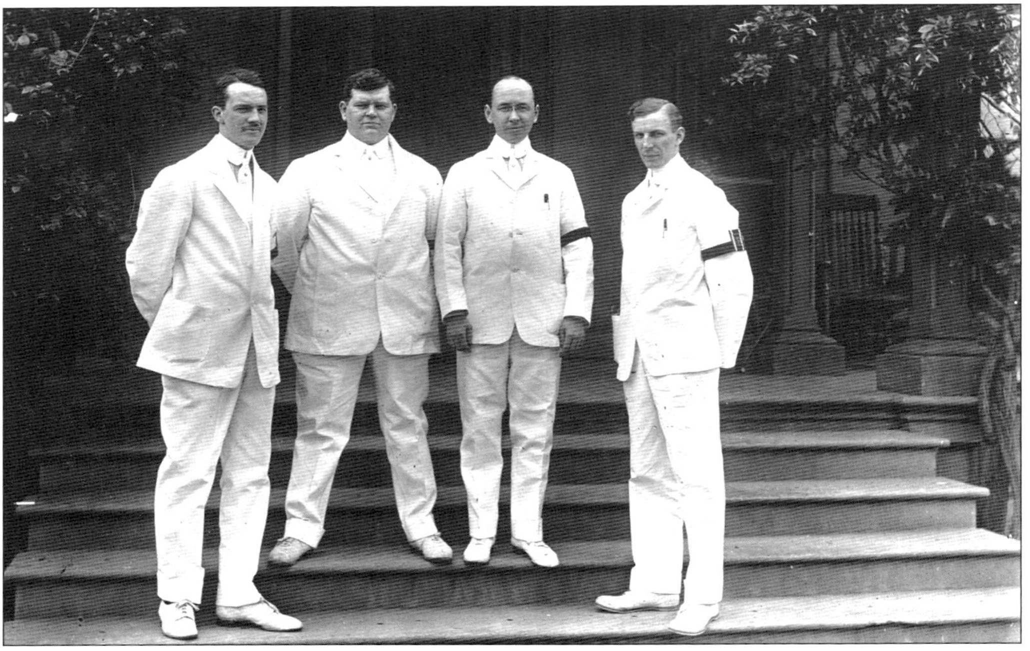

Pictured from left to right, Carlyle N. Haines, George W. Hawk, M. A. Nicholson, and A. M. Loope were assistant physicians in 1912.

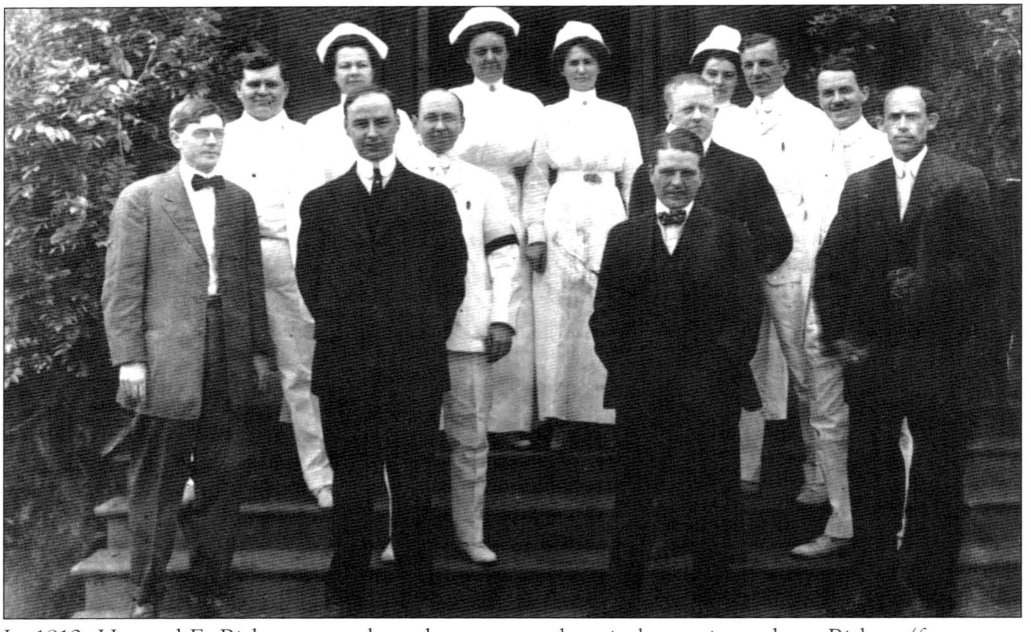

In 1912, Howard E. Bishop was selected to serve as hospital superintendent. Bishop (front row, far left) is pictured with the following Robert Packer Hospital staff, from left to right, (first row) Dr. Silas Molyneux, Dr. Donald Guthrie, and X-ray operator and photographer A. T. Weaver; (second row) Dr. George W. Hawk, Dr. Rufus Reeves, Dr. Walter E. Lundblad, Dr. Phillip Schwartz, and Dr. C. N. Haines; (third row) nurses Margaret Ohlman, Cleo Hollopeter, Julia Coyle, and Belle Spencer.

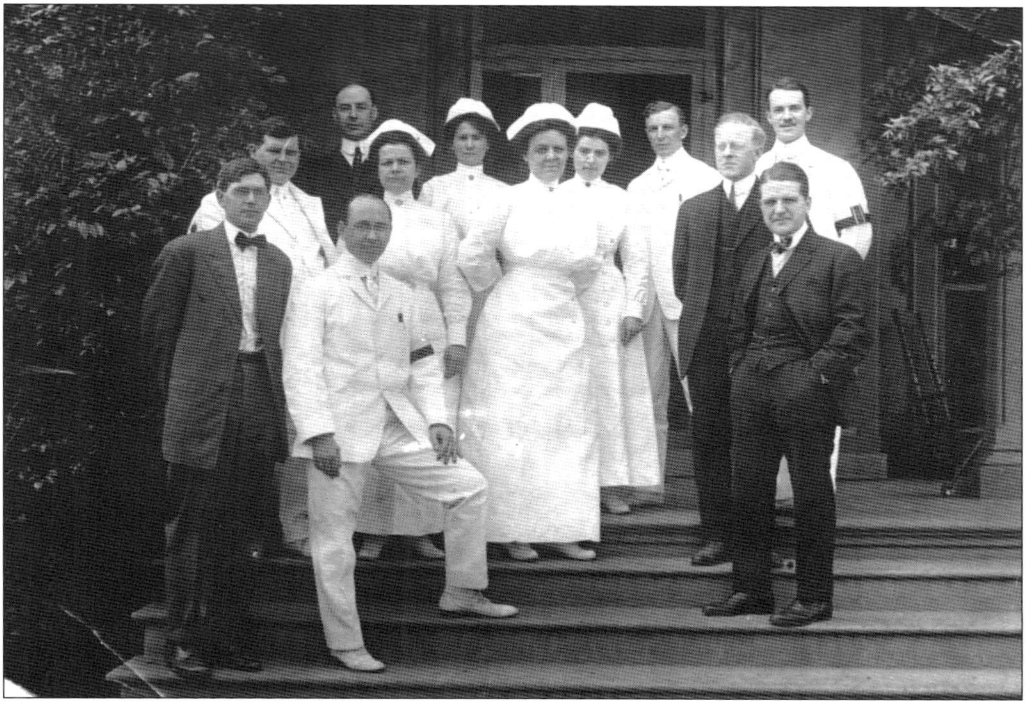

A photograph of Robert Packer Hospital staff in 1913 shows the following staff, from left to right: (first row) administrator Howard E. Bishop, Dr. Rufus Green, and Dr. Donald Guthrie; (second row) Dr. George W. Hawk, Margaret Ohlman, directress of nurses Cleo Hollopeter, and Dr. Walter E. Lundblad; (third row) Dr. Silas Molyneux, operating room nurse Julia Coyle, anesthetist Belle Spencer, Dr. Phillip Schwartz, and Dr. Carlyle N. Haines.

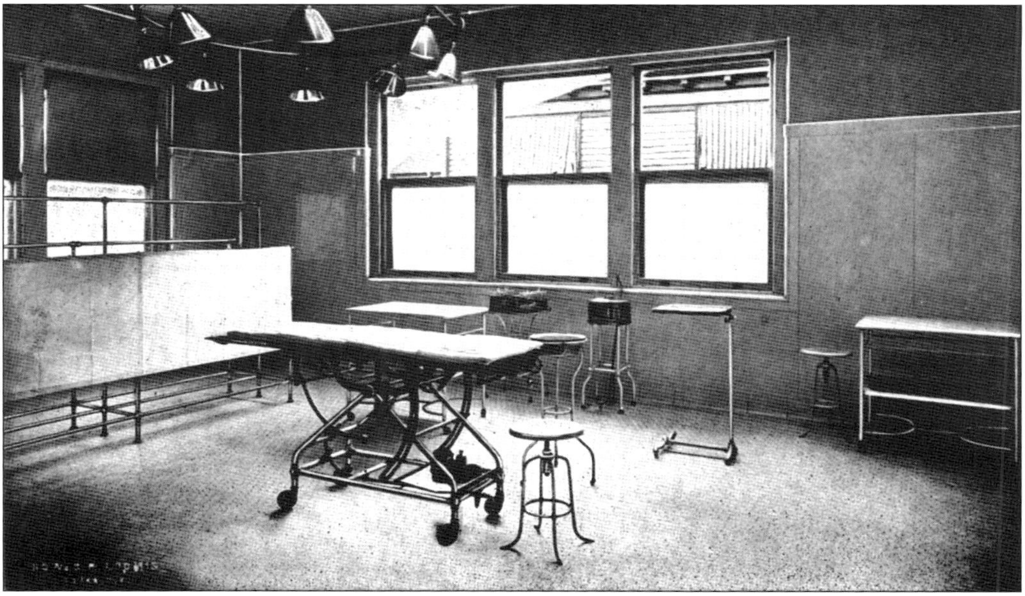

The west operating room of the Dr. Ott Memorial Pavilion opened to the public on December 16, 1913.

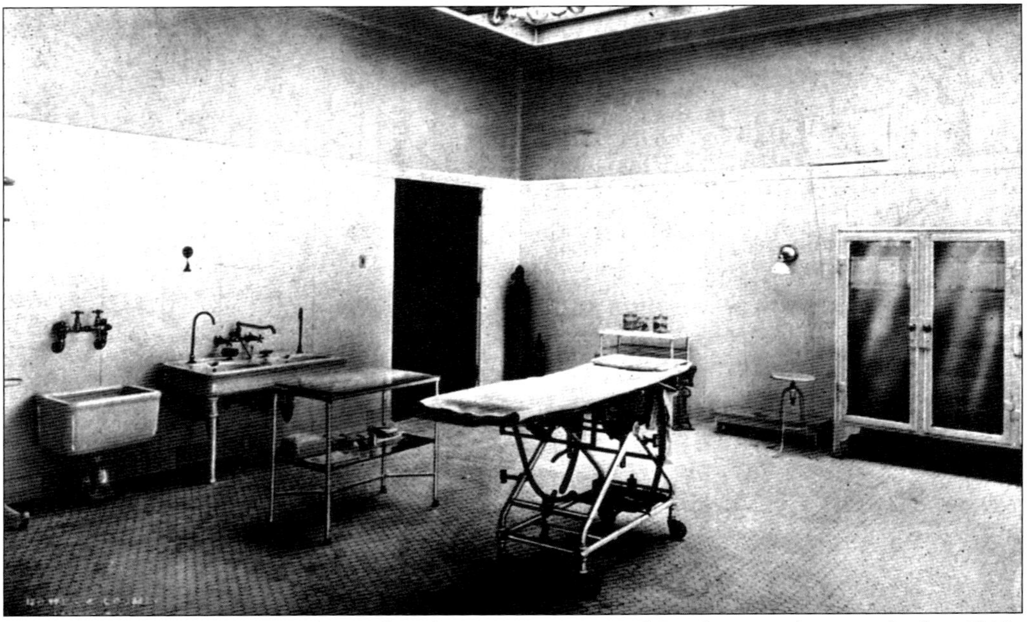

The east operating room was located in the Dr. Ott Memorial Pavilion, as photographed in 1914.

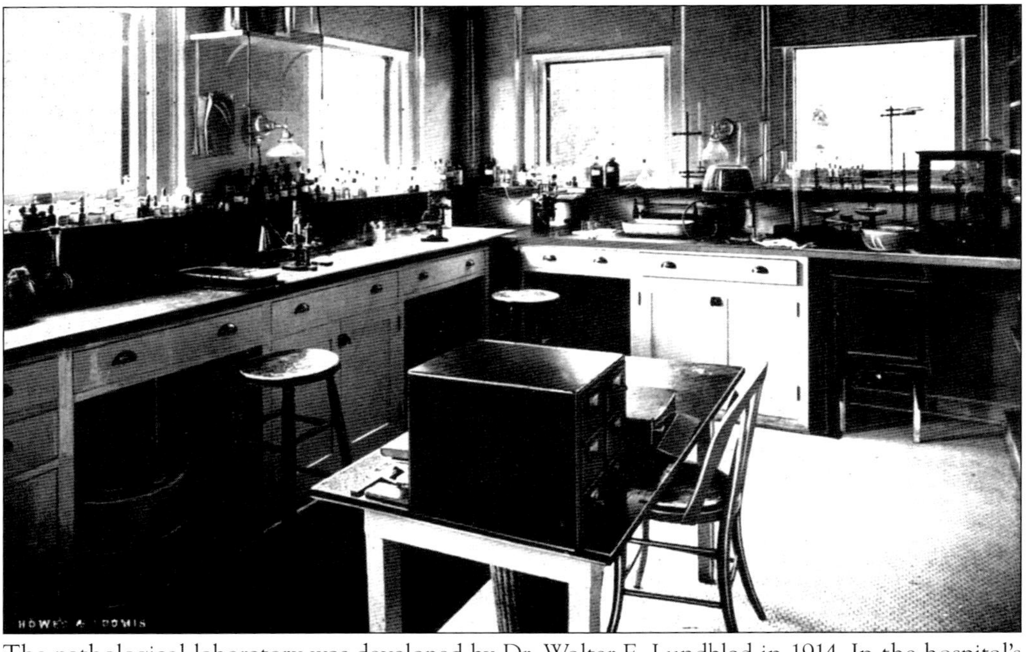

The pathological laboratory was developed by Dr. Walter E. Lundblad in 1914. In the hospital's annual report for that year, Dr. Donald Guthrie stated, "The pathological department which is the greatest help to us in our work is being used more and more by physicians locally and from a distance."

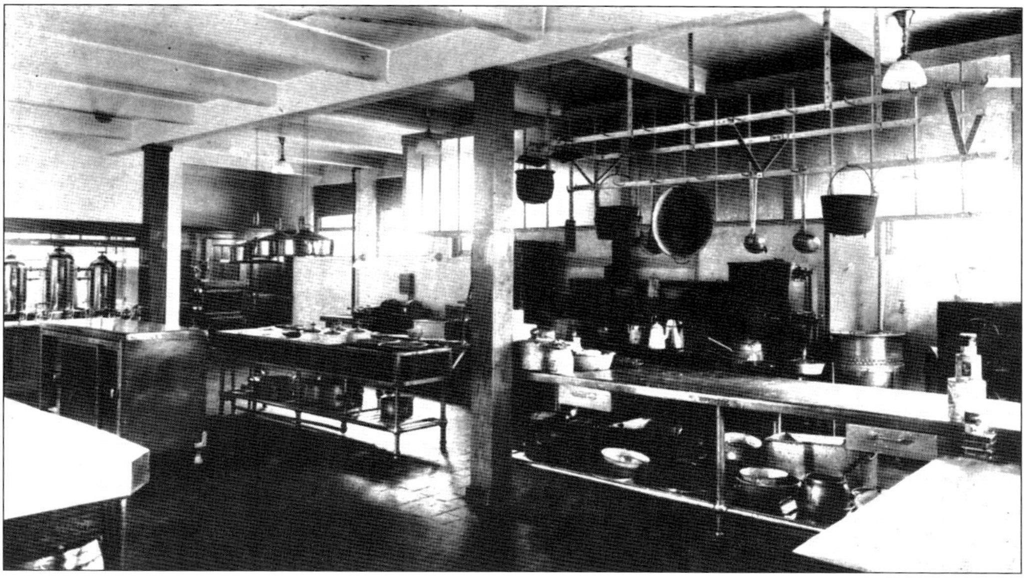

The main kitchen, constructed in a fireproof building in 1915, was completed in the middle of January and put right to use. Supt. Howard E. Bishop said, "I am sure we have made no mistake in expending a large amount of money in this department, which next to the operating pavilion is the most important part of our whole institution."

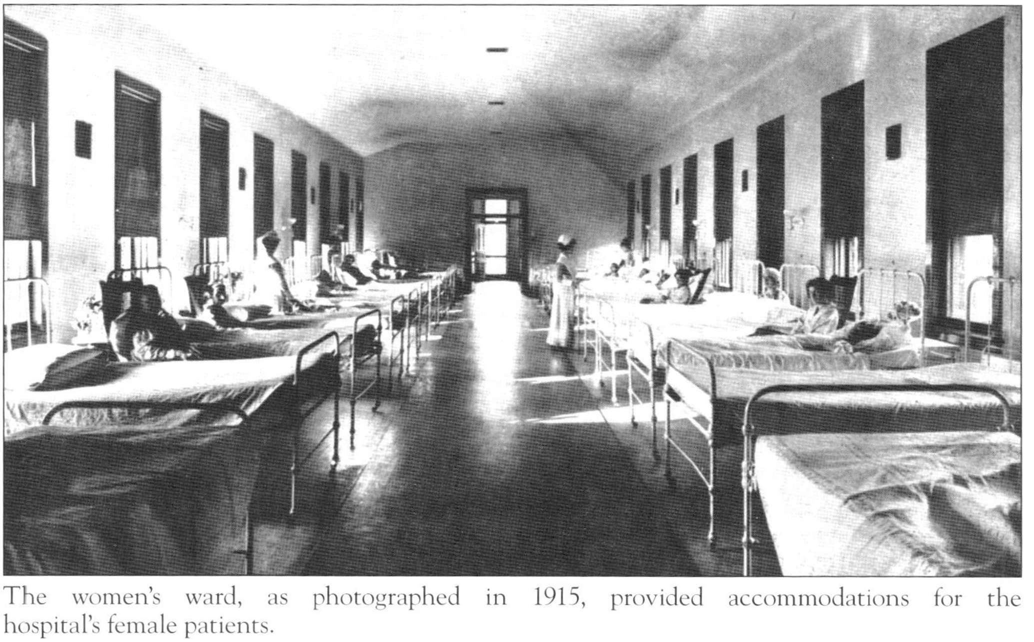

The women's ward, as photographed in 1915, provided accommodations for the hospital's female patients.

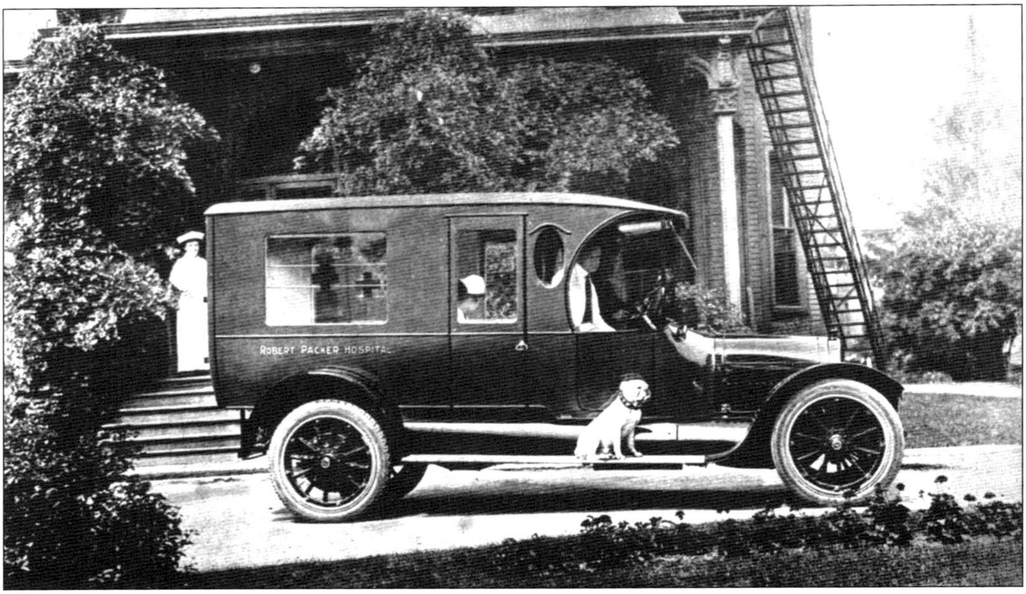

In 1916, C. H. Jennings and W. W. Jennings provided the hospital with a new ambulance. In this photograph, Dr. Donald Guthrie's dog Rip Van Winkle tries out the vehicle's running board.

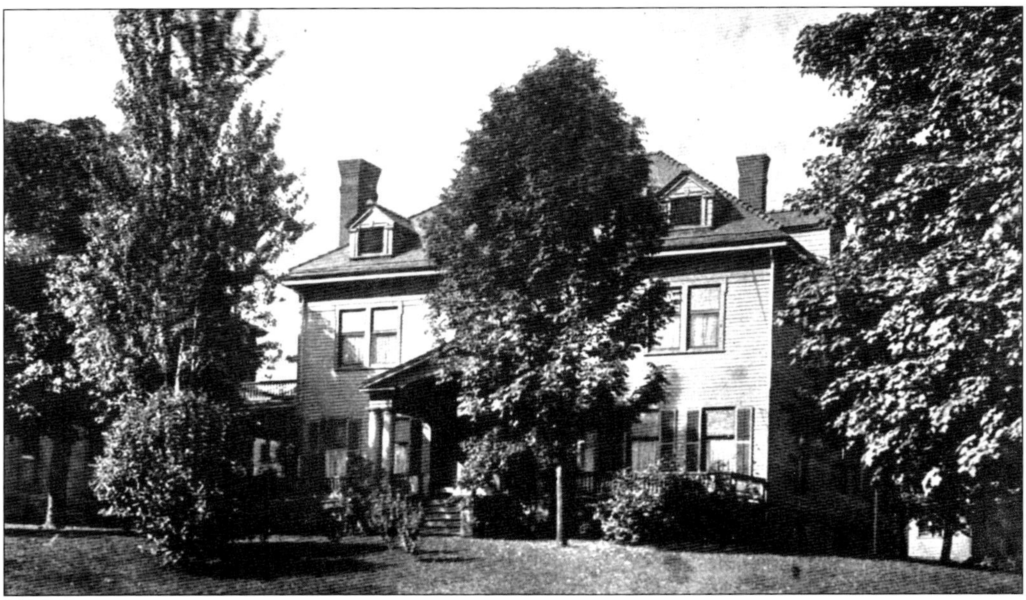

The surgeon's residence stood beside Packer Mansion, as shown in this photograph from 1916. Today part of the Patterson Education Building occupies this lot.

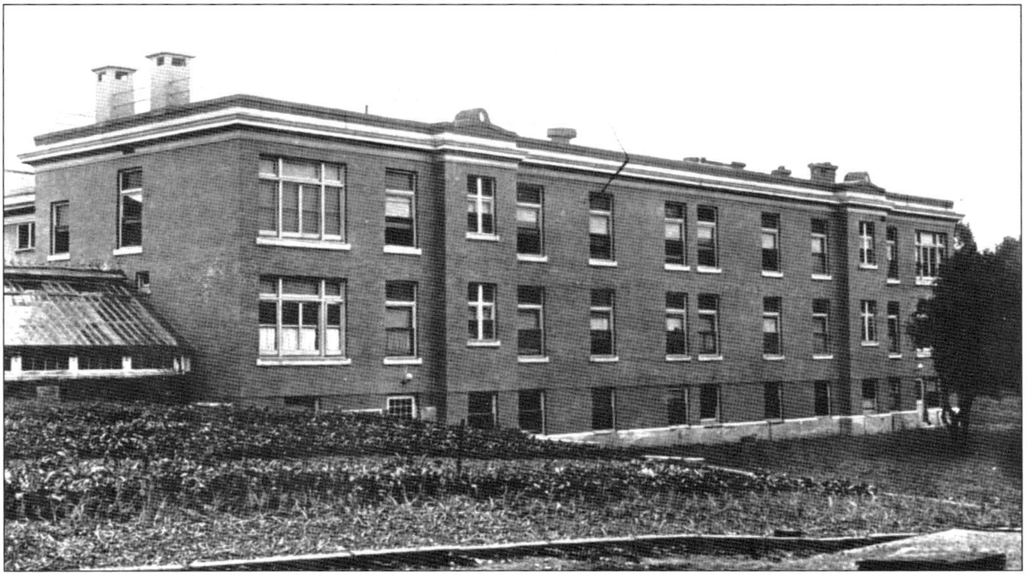

The private rooms pavilion opened in 1917. Dr. Guthrie said of the new facility, "The wisdom of building a new private rooms pavilion has been fully demonstrated for the rooms have been in demand. In fact twice since it opened last January every room has been taken."

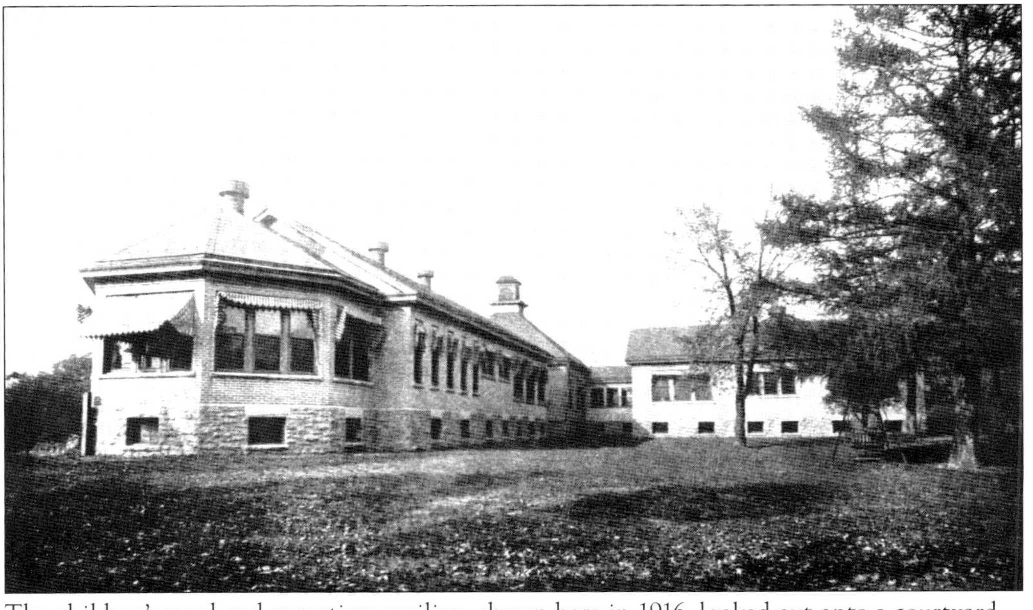

The children's ward and operating pavilion, shown here in 1916, looked out onto a courtyard.

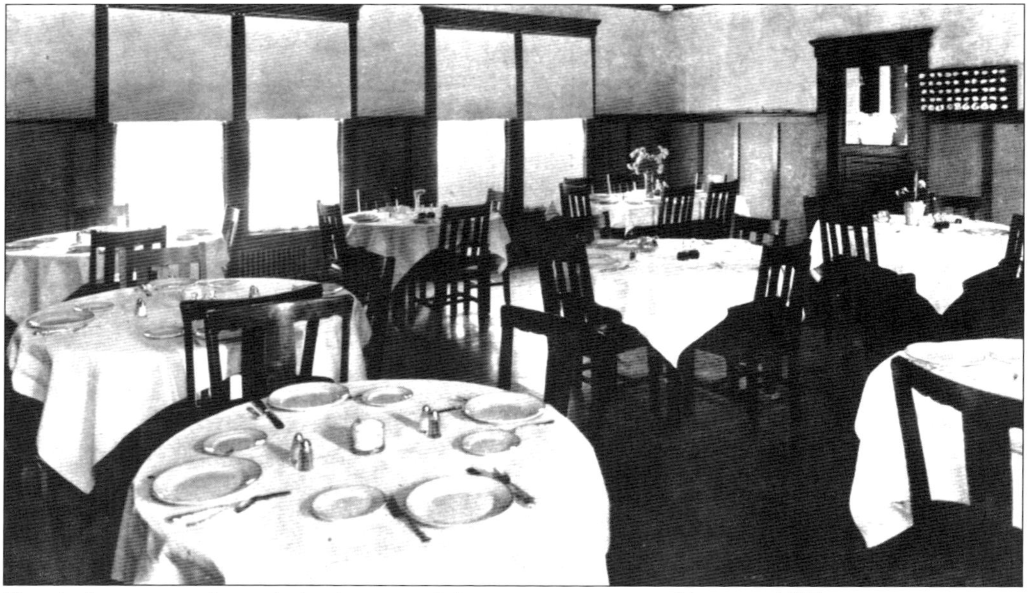

Hospital nurses took meals in the nurses' dining room, pictured here in 1915.

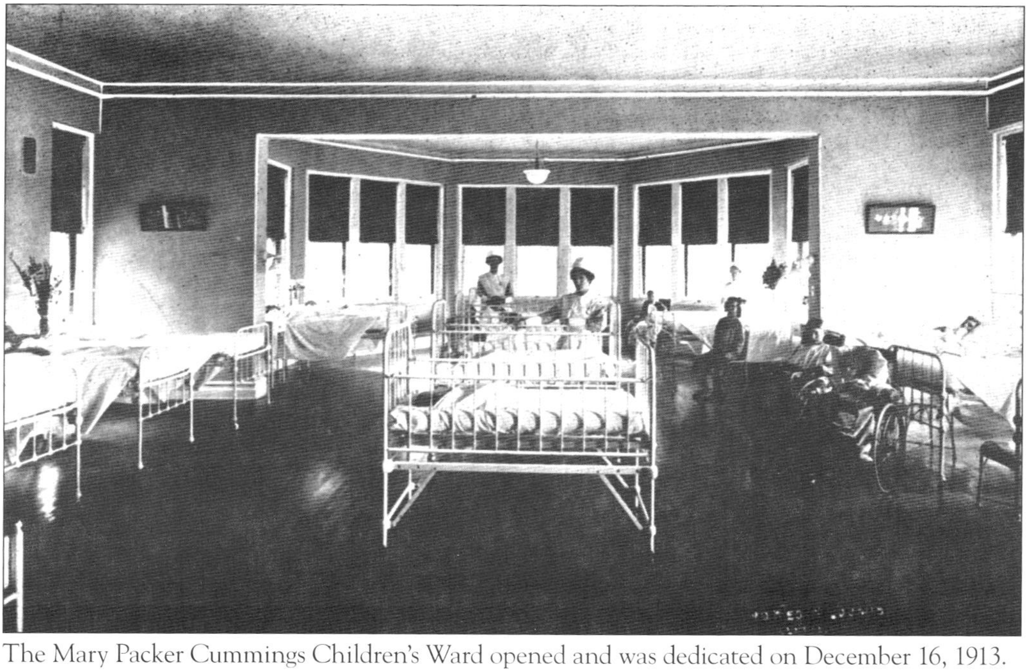

The Mary Packer Cummings Children's Ward opened and was dedicated on December 16, 1913.

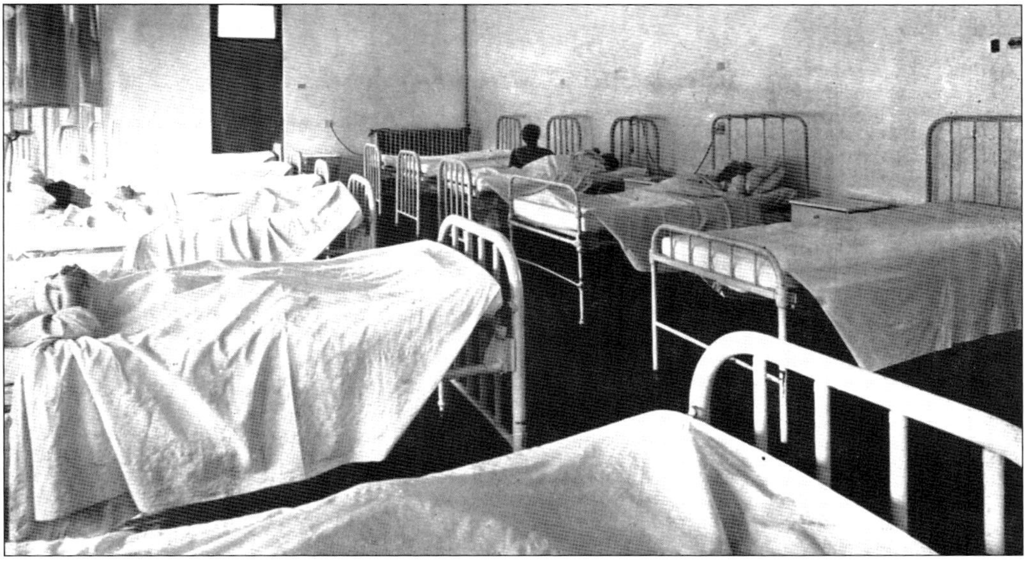

The women's sun ward, shown in this picture taken in 1917, provided female patients with access to sunlight, which was considered a beneficial treatment for some illnesses.

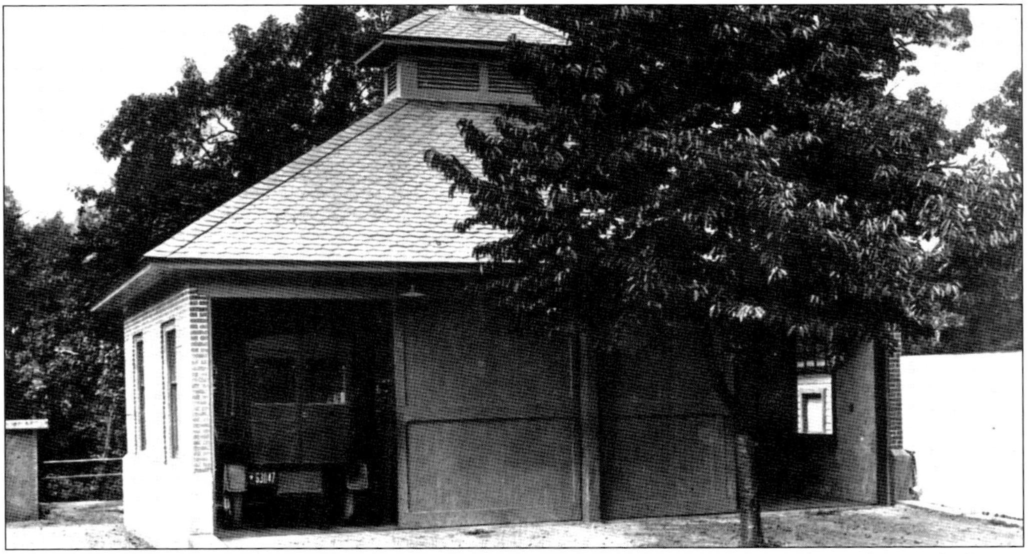

A new garage was built of brick and concrete in 1917 to accommodate the ambulance and three cars.

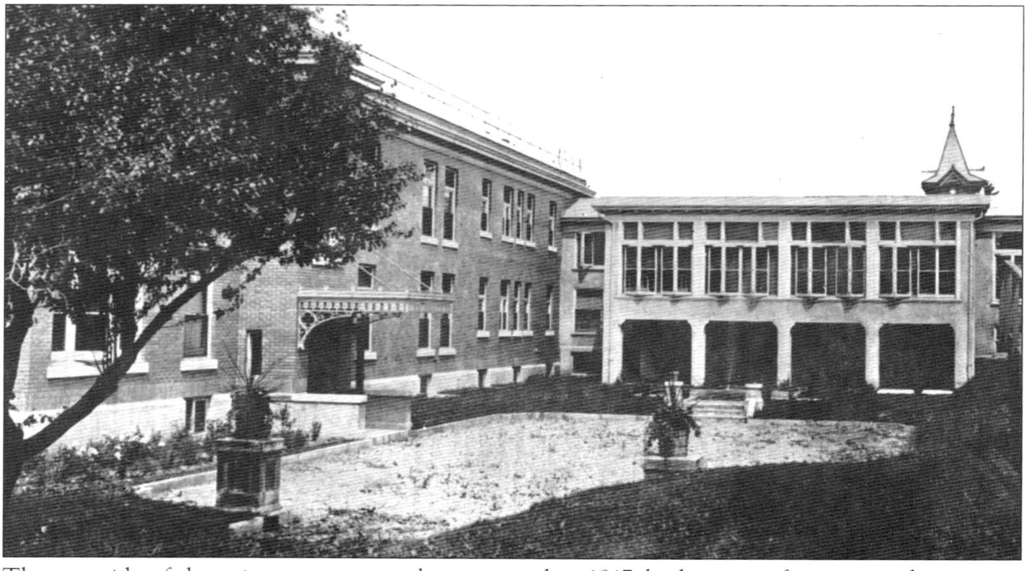

The east side of the private rooms pavilion, opened in 1917, had a view of a courtyard.

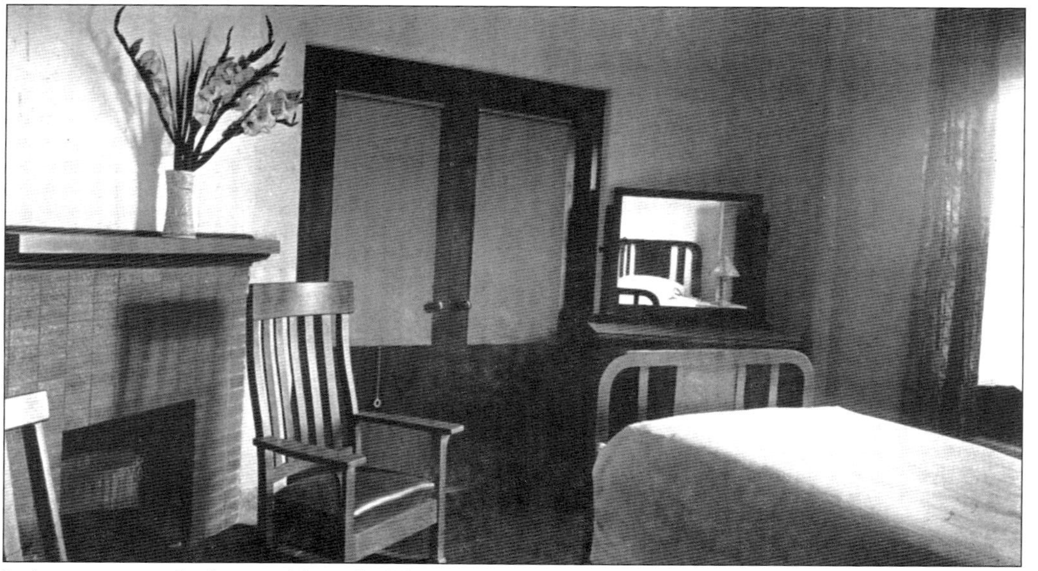

In his report to the hospital board of directors in 1917, Dr. Donald Guthrie described the private rooms pavilion's accommodations as "beautifully furnished and appointed."

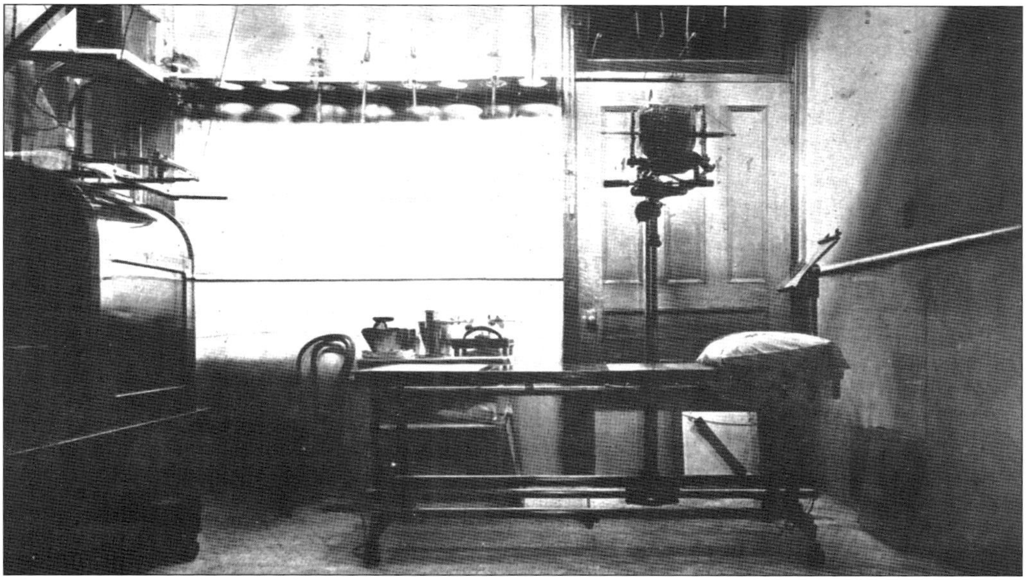

This photograph shows early radiology equipment in the hospital's X-ray room in 1919.

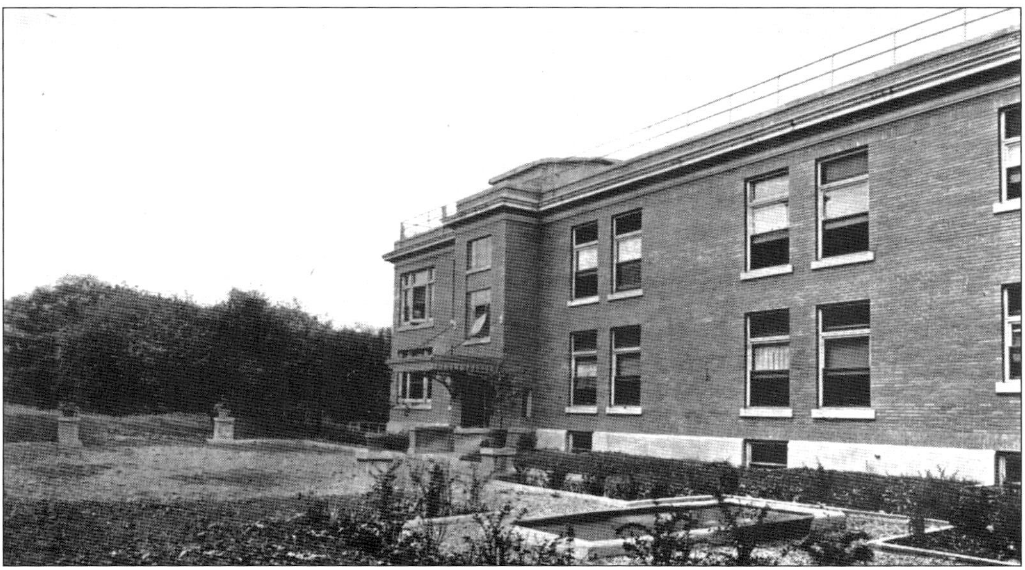

The hospital included an obstetrical pavilion, which is pictured here in 1918.

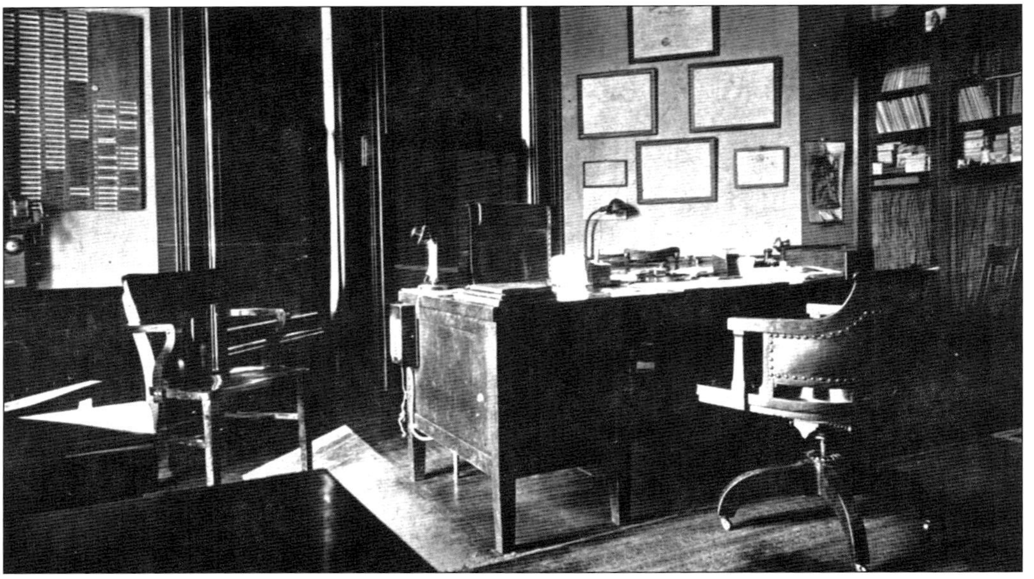

The superintendent's office, shown around 1919, was located in Packer Mansion.

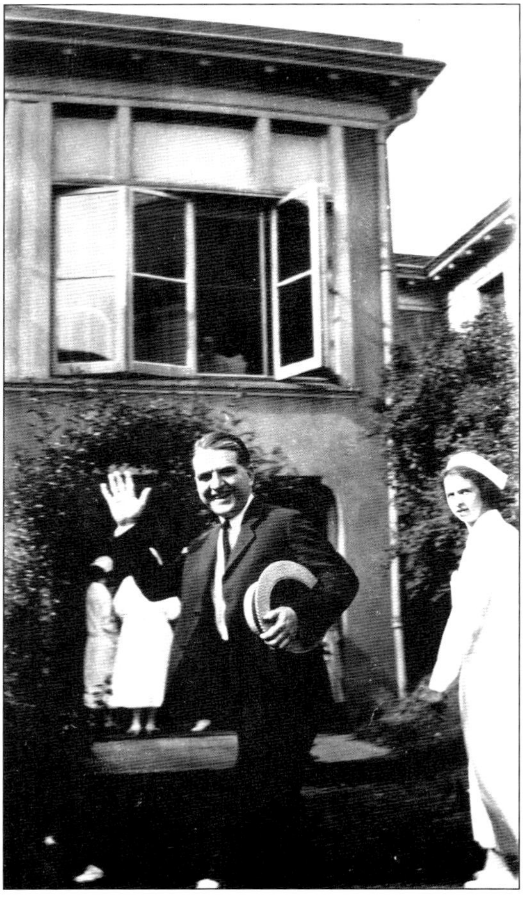

Dr. Donald Guthrie was photographed passing through the courtyard near the private rooms pavilion in 1912.

Four

THE CLINIC AND HOSPITAL CONTINUE TO GROW

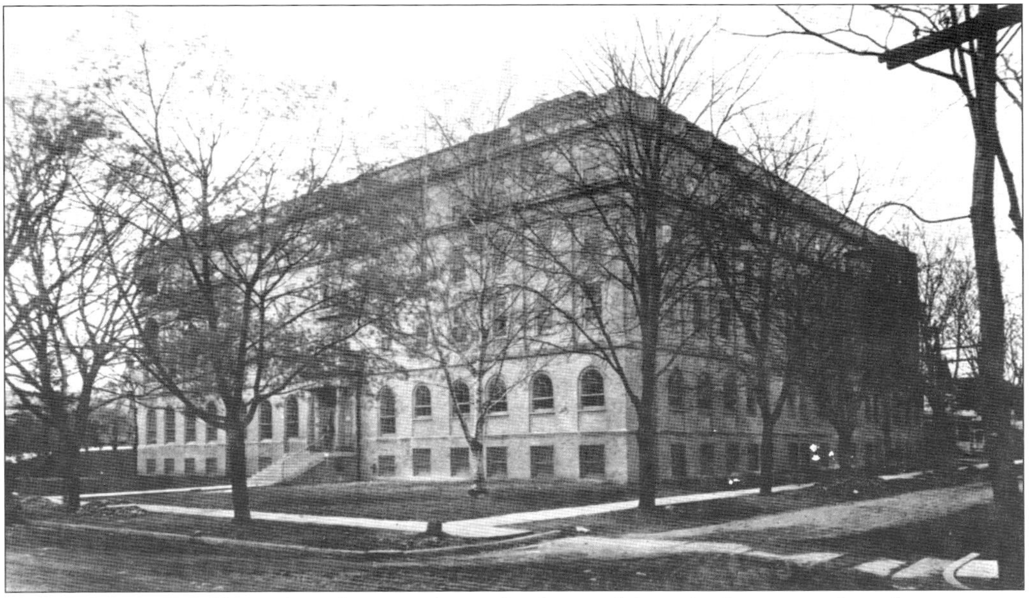

In 1920, Dr. Donald Guthrie began asking the hospital board of trustees for a larger, more modern school of nursing and clinic buildings. By the end of the decade, both new buildings were constructed and in use. Dr. Guthrie had four requirements for health care: the primary focus must always be the welfare of the patient; the emphasis must always lean toward care; continuing education is a necessity for the physician, nurses, and technicians; and research must provide benefits applicable to the care of the sick. All the new construction and improvements were in line with these requirements.

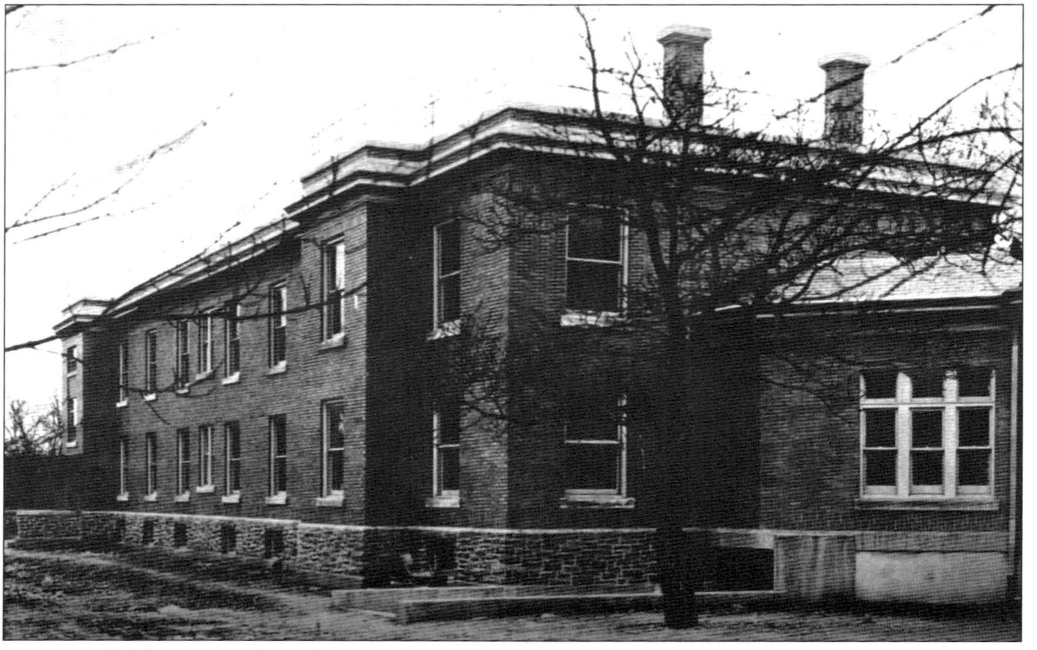

A new children's ward and maternity building was constructed in 1921 and opened on January 1, 1922. The cost of the building was $86,065.

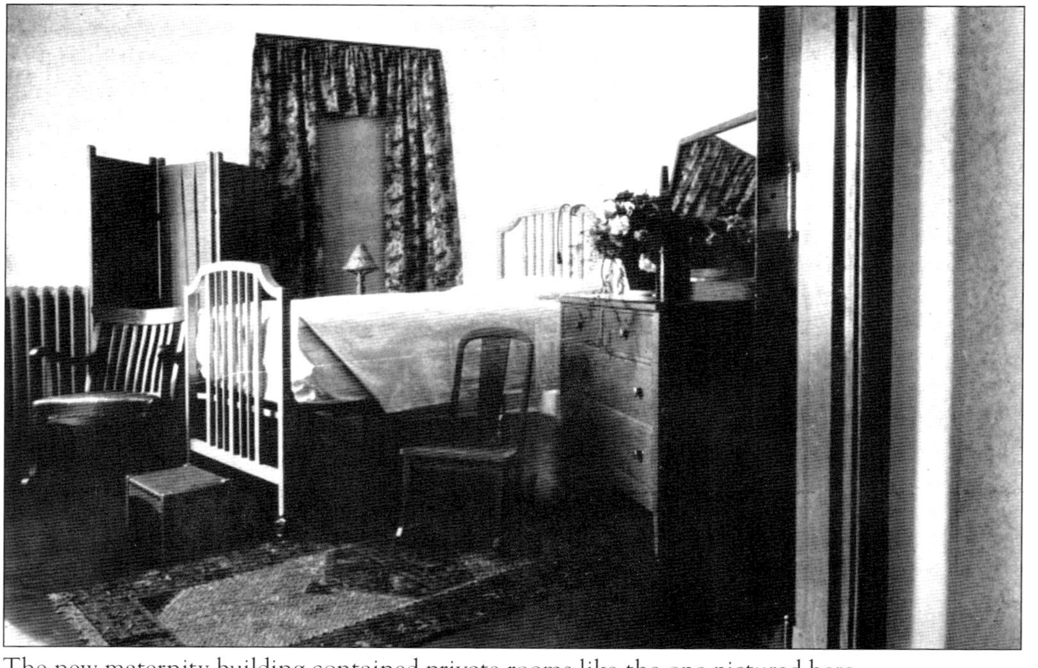

The new maternity building contained private rooms like the one pictured here.

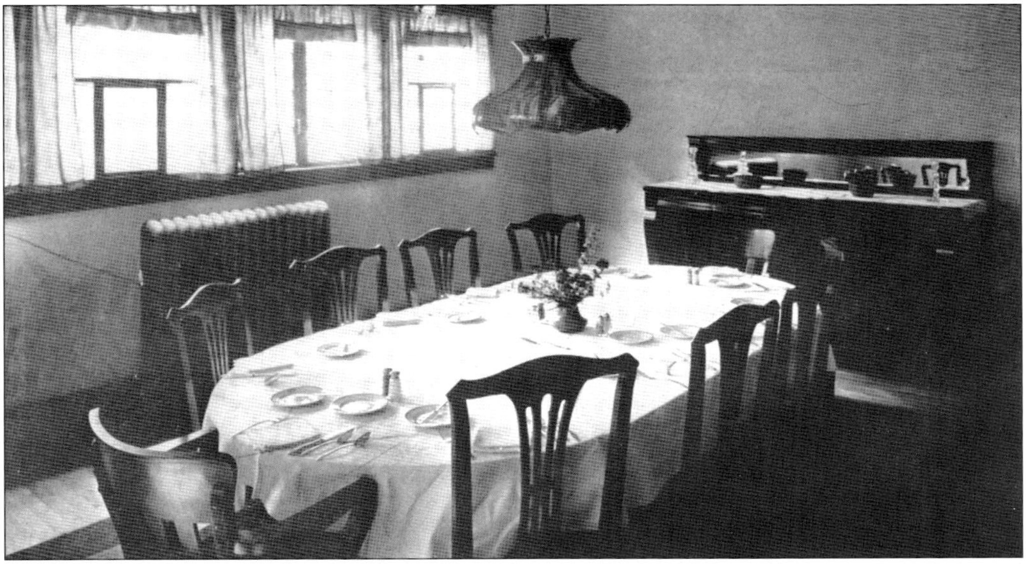

The hospital's physicians made good use of the private doctors' dining room, pictured here in 1921.

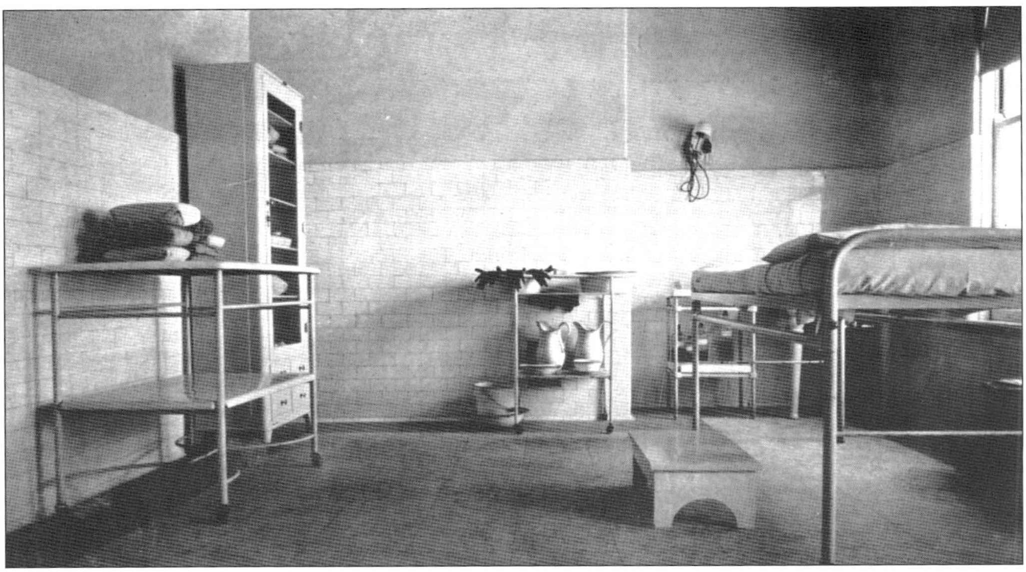

The new maternity building included this delivery room.

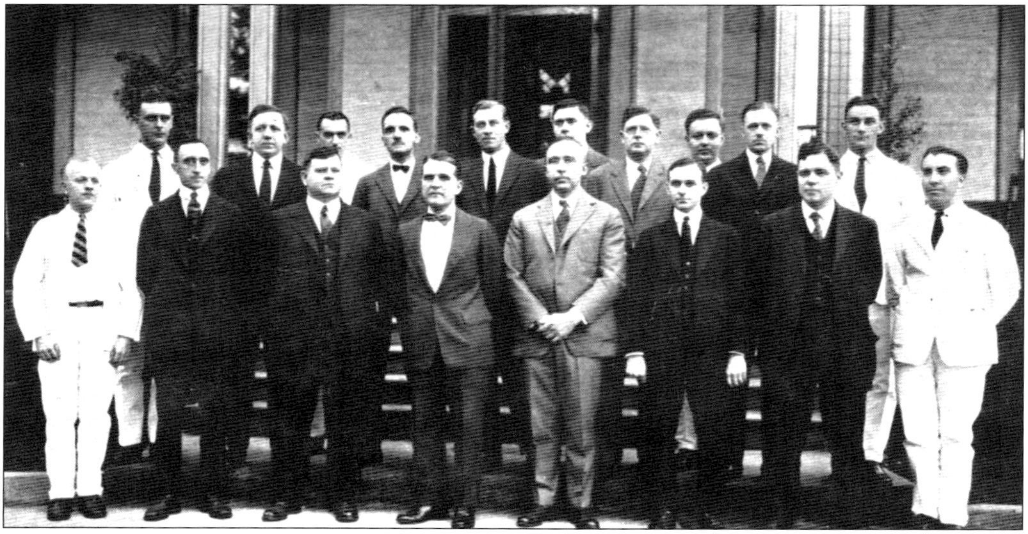

Members of the hospital staff in 1925 are, from left to right, (first row) Dr. J. F. Kleinhecksel, Dr. Charles H. DeWan, Dr. George W. Hawk, Dr. Donald Guthrie, Dr. Nelson S. Weinberger, Dr. Stanley D. Conklin, Dr. John M. Higgins, and Dr. Louis M. Fowler; (second row) Dr. Manville Norton, Dr. Carlyle N. Haines, Dr. M. W. Bodine, X-ray operator Sydney T. Purkiss, Dr. George F. Carling, Dr. Robert C. Murdy, Supt. Howard E. Bishop, Dr. R. DuVal Jones, Dr. Ethan Flag Butler, and Dr. Manning Brown. Drs. Jones, Kleinhecksel, Brown, and Bodine finished their residency at Sayre and went to the Mayo Clinic. Dr. Norton also finished his residency at Sayre and went to a tuberculosis camp in Westchester County, New York.

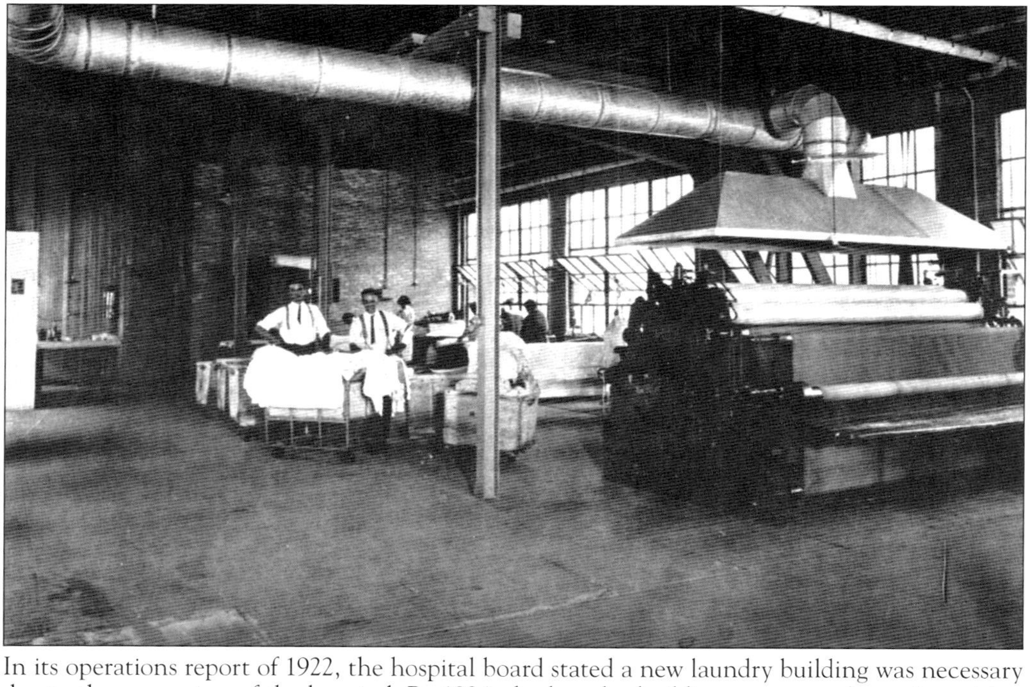

In its operations report of 1922, the hospital board stated a new laundry building was necessary due to the expansion of the hospital. By 1924, the laundry building was up and running with a flat work machine and presses (pictured).

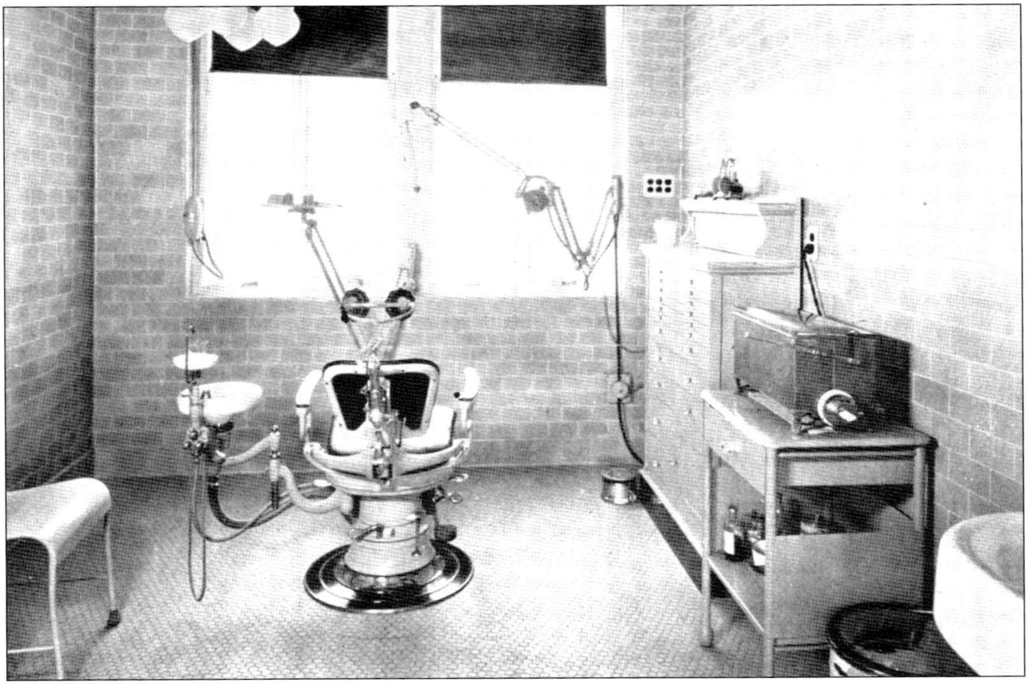

Clinic dentists examined patients and performed surgeries in the dental operating room, as seen in 1926.

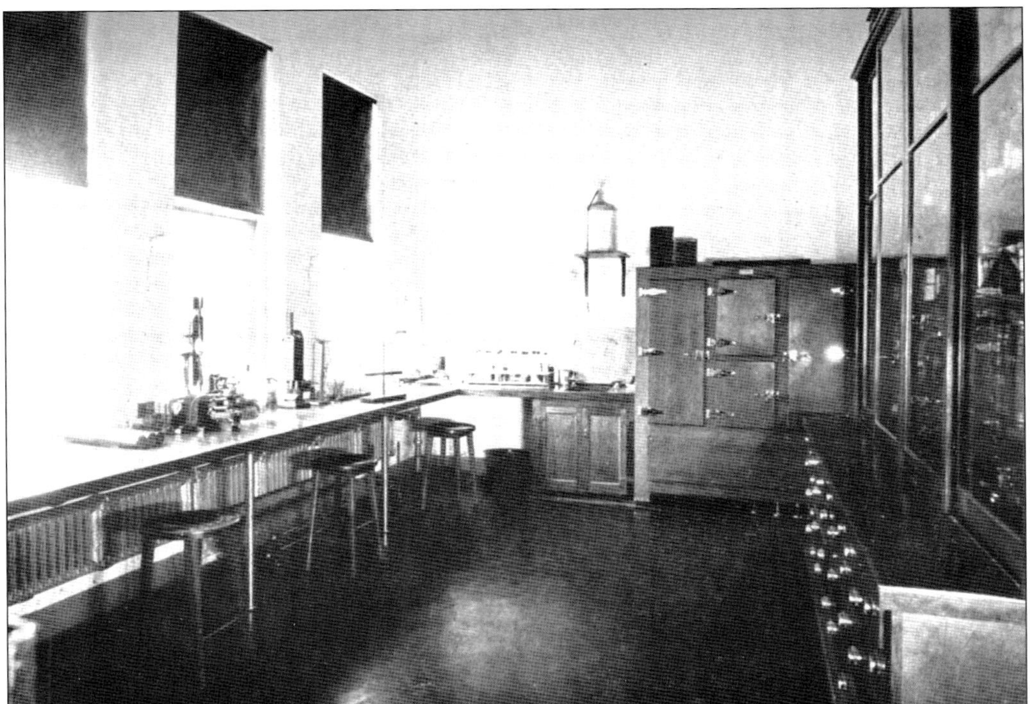

In 1926, the hospital's laboratory staff processed samples in this room.

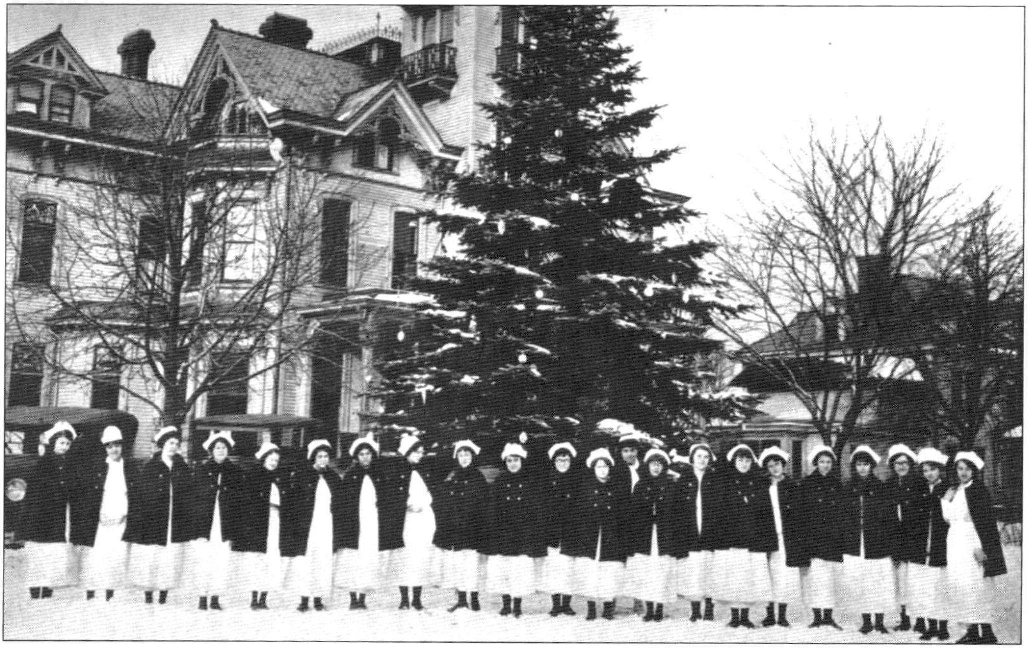

As part of a holiday tradition, the hospital's nurses placed a Christmas tree in front of Packer Mansion, pictured here in 1925.

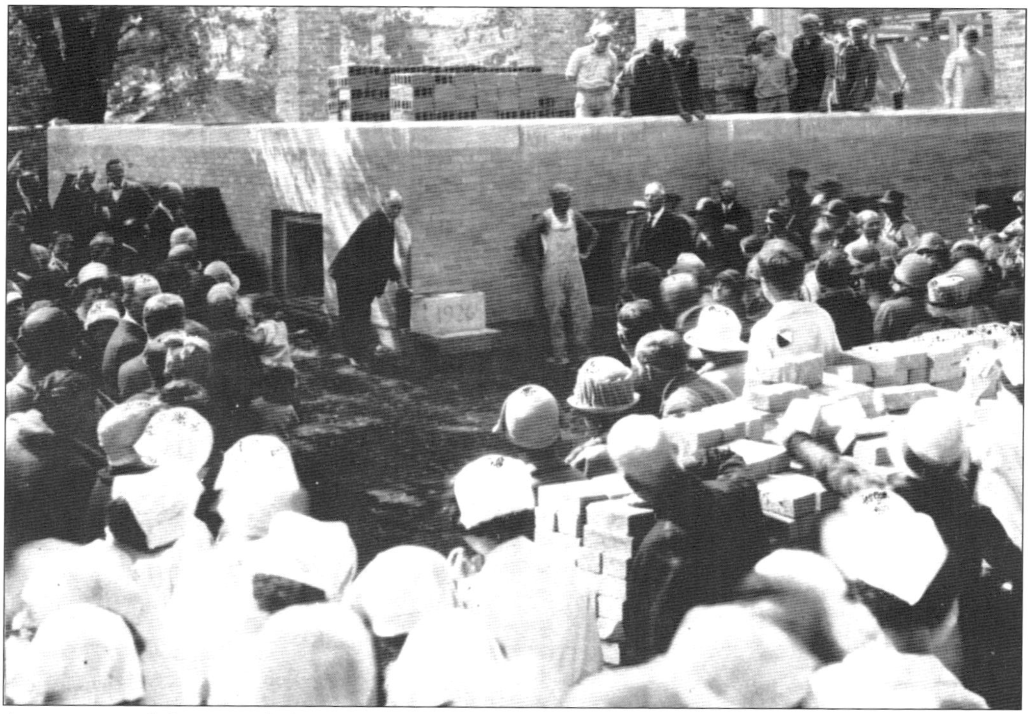

A ceremonial laying of the cornerstone for the nurses' home occurred on June 8, 1926. David A. Keefe of Athens presided over the event. Charles D. Marvin laid the stone. The home was the realization of many years of hopes and plans.

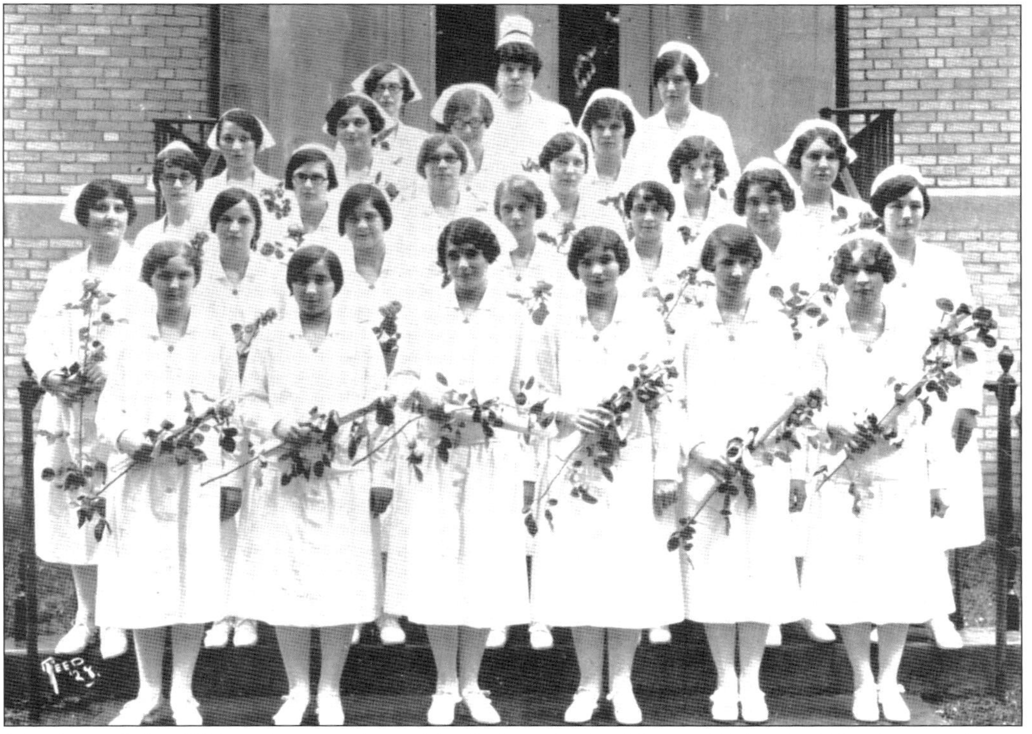

Members of the 1928 graduating class of the Robert Packer Hospital School of Nursing are shown here with Nina A. Smith, RN, directress of nursing (middle of the top row). The graduates are Hazel S. Anderson, Jeannette Baxter, Romaine D. Bowman, Mary M. Cease, Nell G. DePew, Elsie W. Dukett, Simie L. Eskeli, Kathleen S. Francis, Helen M. Gooding, Katheryn L. Hess, Julia Hopkins, Frances C. Huffmaster, Monica M. Hurley, Myra A. Jackman, Mame A. Kump, Evelyn T. Marison, Dorothy L. Neal, Lydia G. Packard, Pauline B. Platt, Ida E. Powers, Lillian E. Rockefeller, Velma F. Scouten, Evelyn A. Tompkins, Julia M. York, and Elizabeth A. Young.

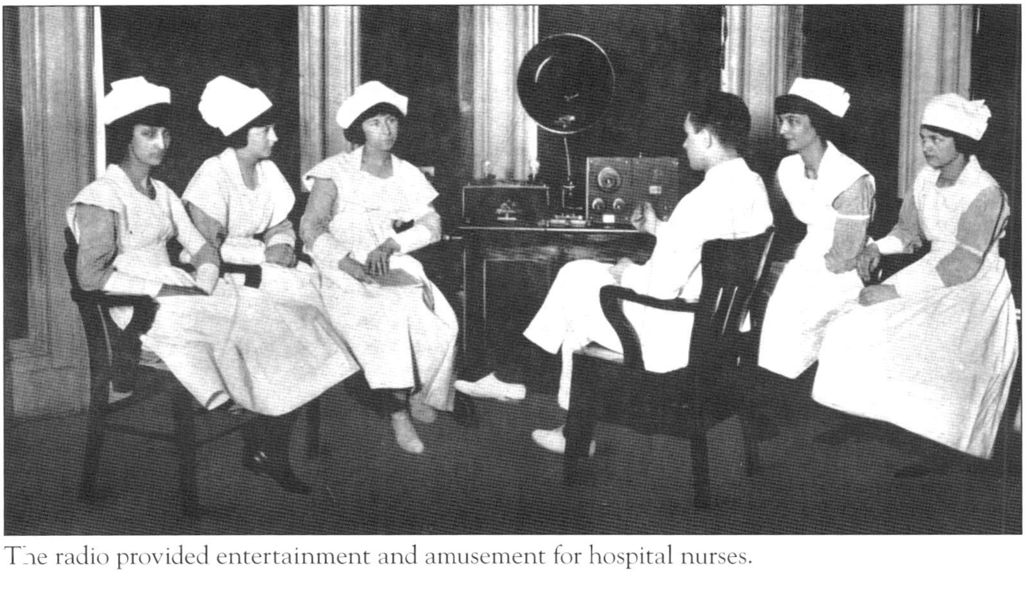

The radio provided entertainment and amusement for hospital nurses.

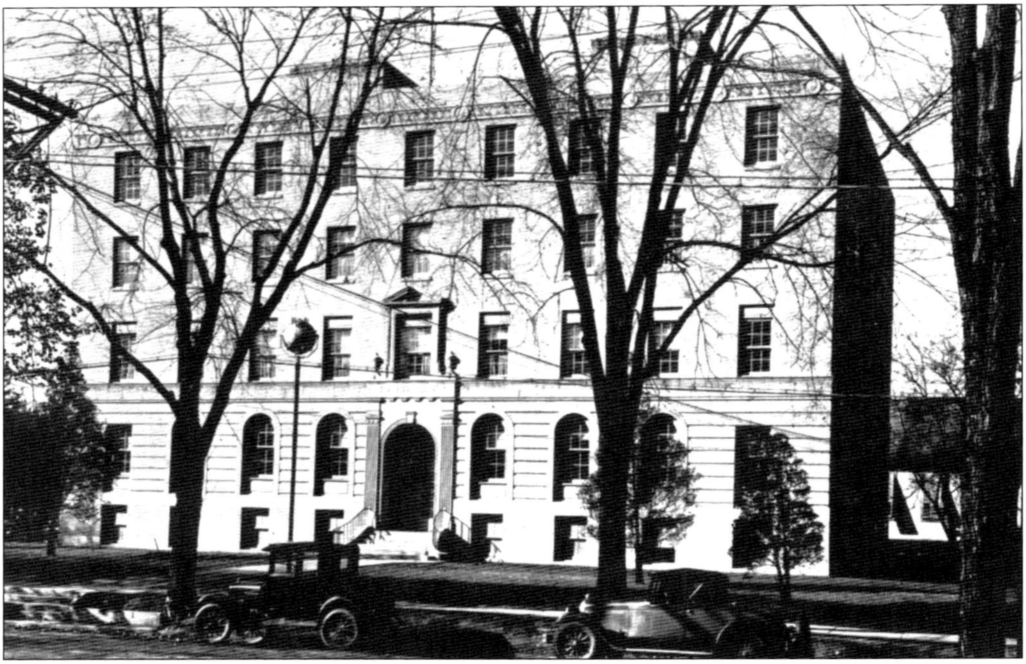

Built in 1927 and 1928, Guthrie Clinic was occupied on December 1, 1928. The building and furnishings cost $300,000. Prior to the building's construction, all work was done in the overcrowded hospital. Dr. Donald Guthrie felt patient care was sometimes compromised by these conditions.

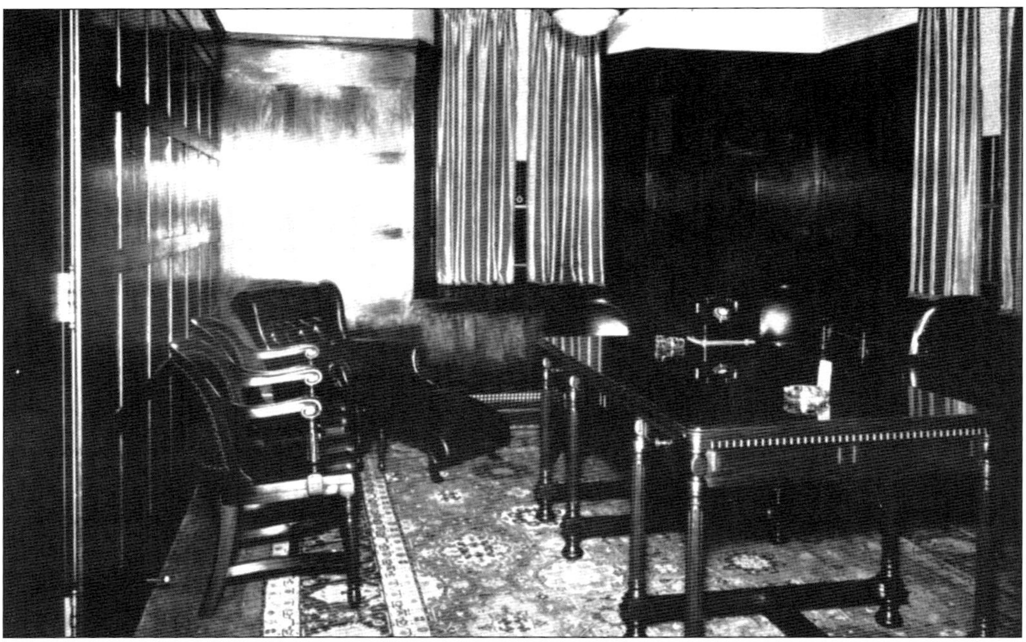

Dr. Guthrie had a private conference room in the clinic building completed in 1928.

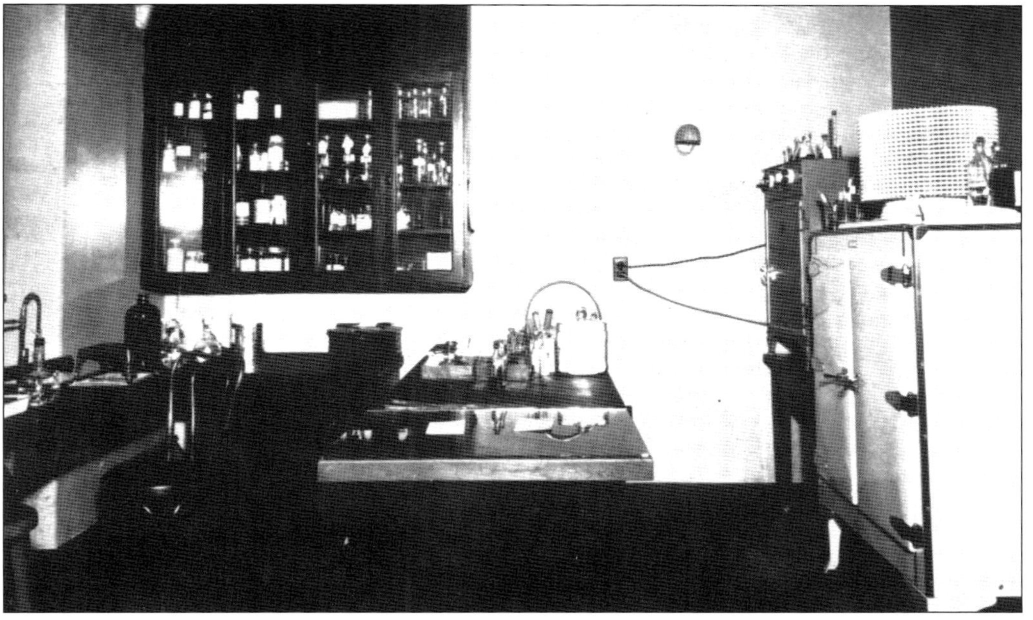

The clinic building included a bacteriological laboratory, pictured here in 1929.

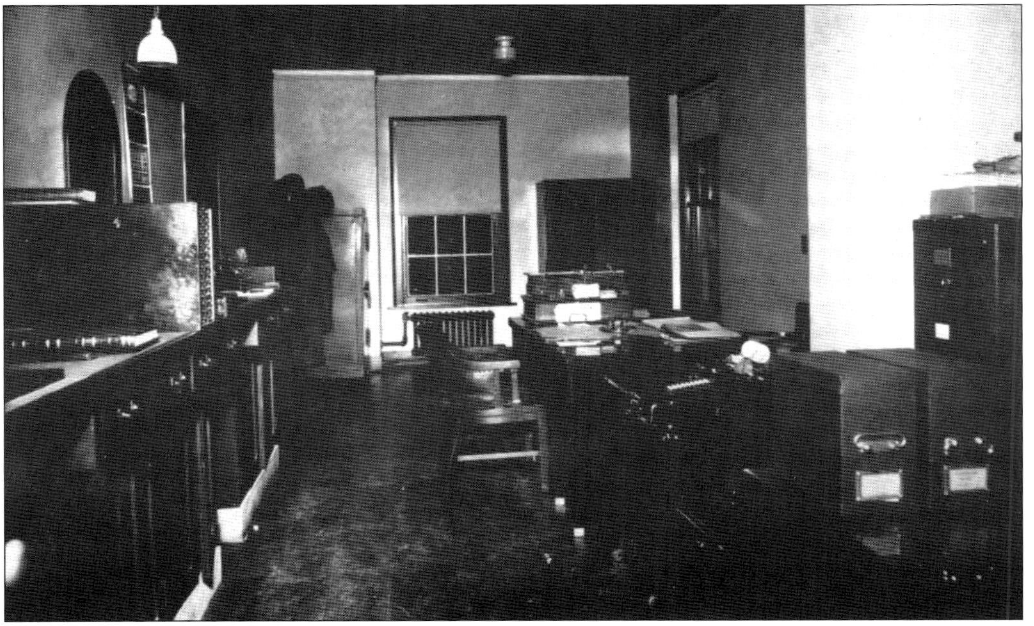

Shown is the Guthrie Clinic business office as it looked in 1928 when the clinic building opened.

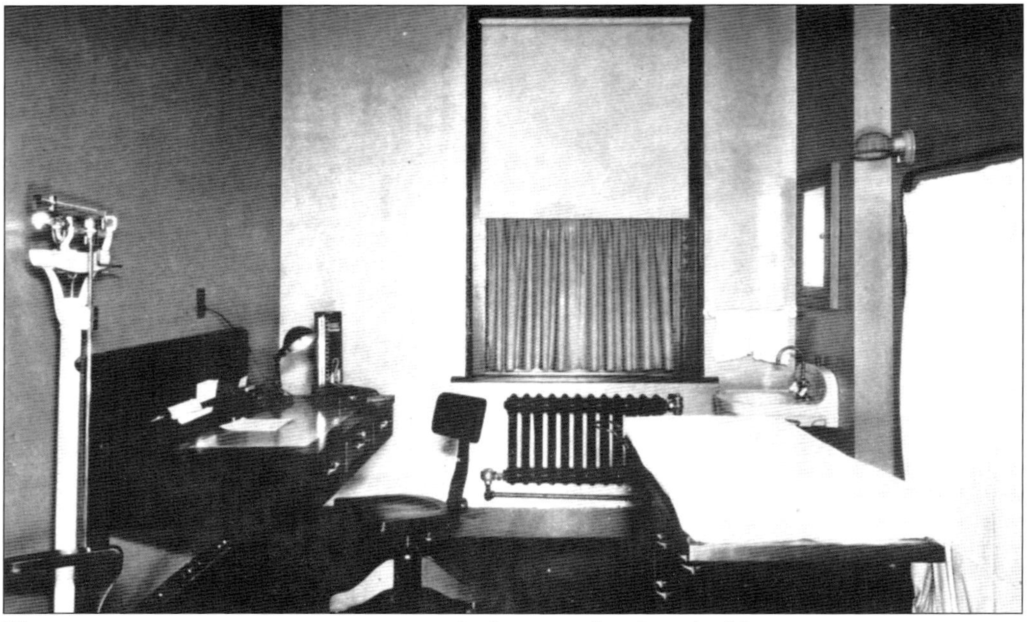

This patient examination room was typical of ones in the clinic building.

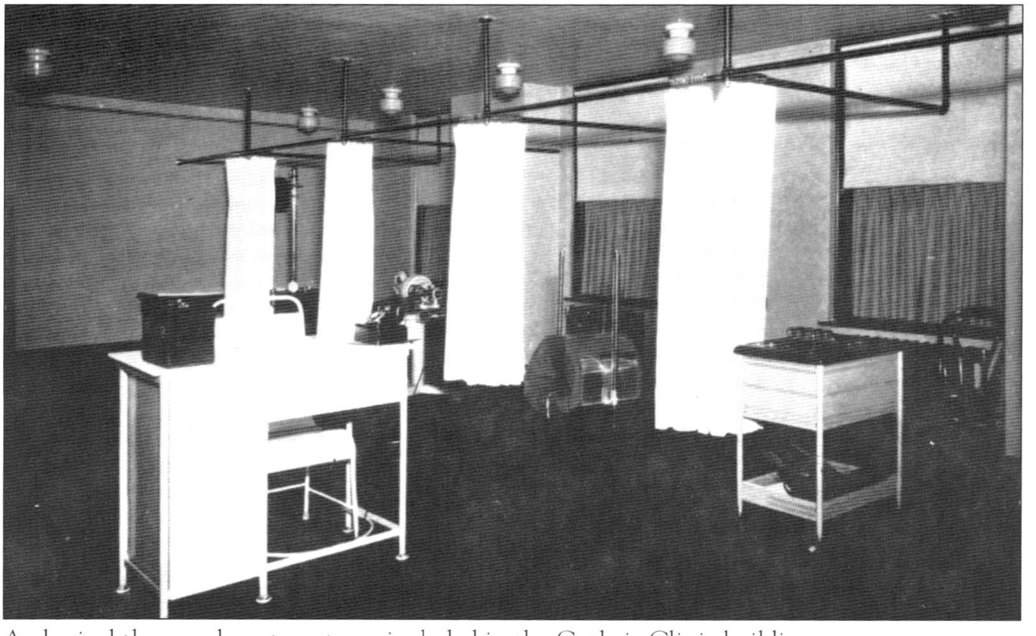

A physical therapy department was included in the Guthrie Clinic building.

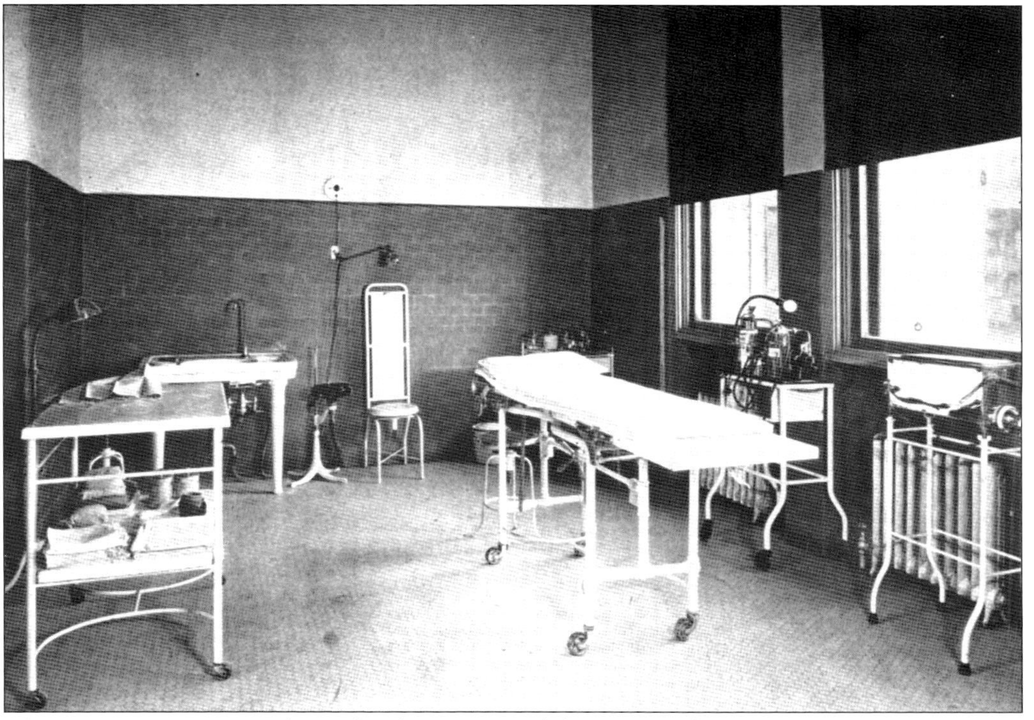
This operating room was devoted only to nose and throat procedures.

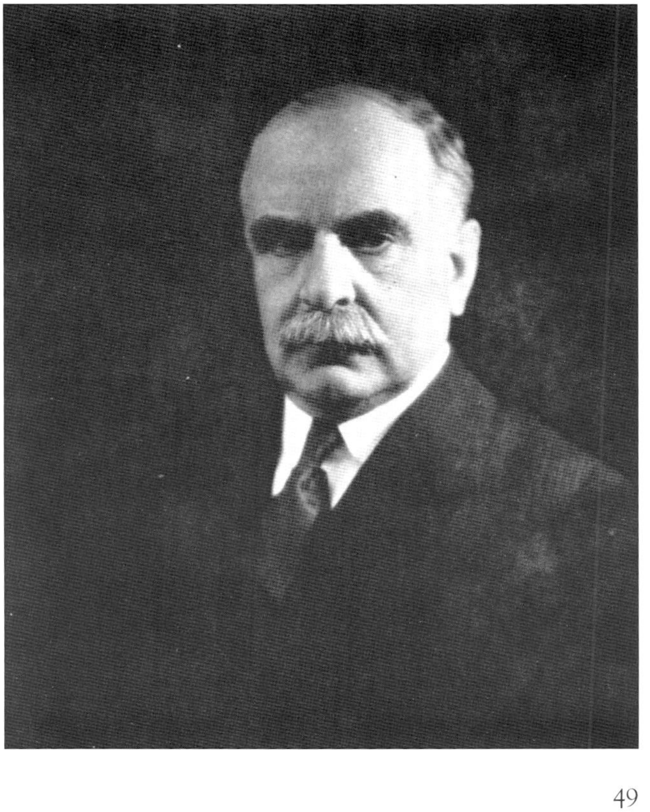
Charles D. Marvin of Owego, New York, was the largest individual contributor to the school of nursing building and the Guthrie Clinic building projects.

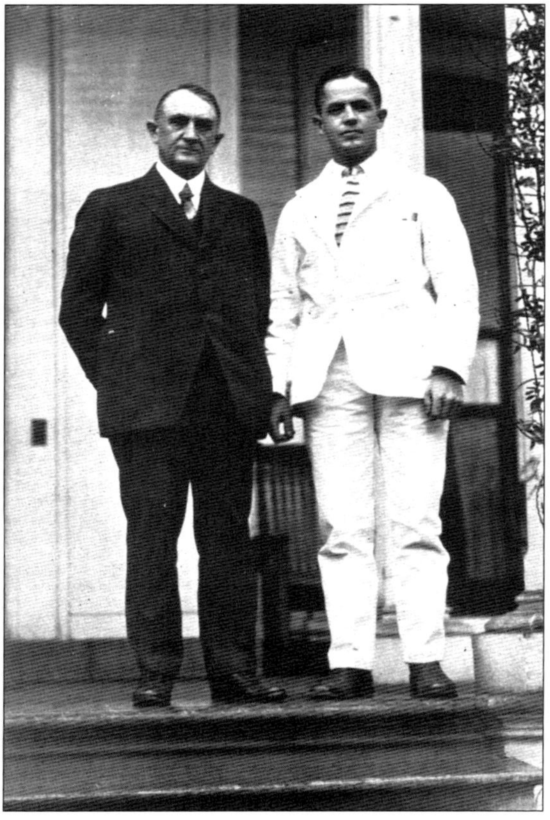

Dr. Charles H. Mayo (left) selected Robert Packer Hospital for the surgical training of his son, Dr. Charles W. Mayo, photographed here in Sayre in 1926. In his report to the board in 1927, Dr. Donald Guthrie said, "I would be a poor historian were I to overlook the honor paid the Robert Packer Hospital by Dr. Charles H. Mayo in selecting this hospital for his son to serve his internship."

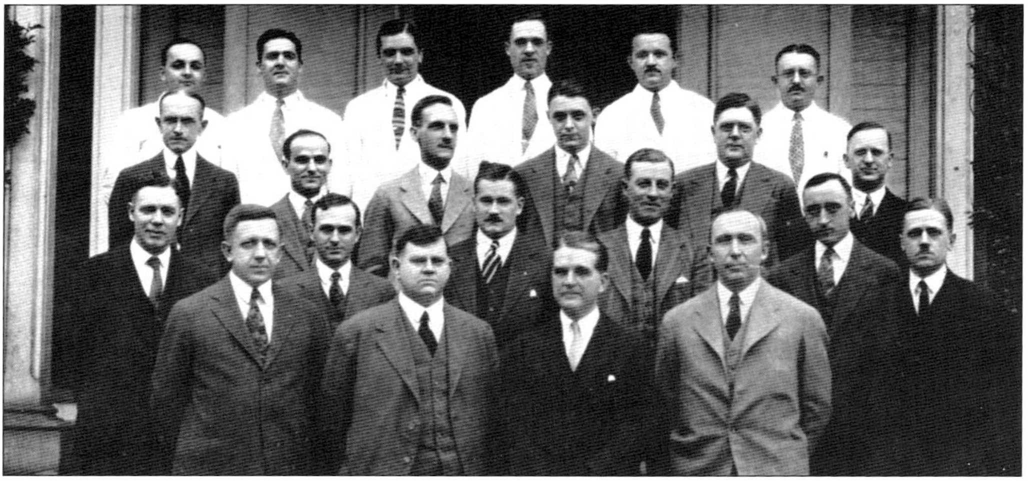

Members of the Robert Packer Hospital staff in 1928 are, from left to right, (first row) Dr. Carlyle N. Haines, Dr. George W. Hawk, Dr. Donald Guthrie, Dr. Nelson S. Weinberger, and Dr. Ethan Flagg Butler; (second row) Dr. John M. Higgins, Dr. Stanley D. Conklin, Dr. Ronald L. Hamilton, Dr. George F. Carling, and Dr. Charles H. DeWan; (third row) Dr. James W. Brice, Dr. Thomas Dimitroff, Sydney T. Purkiss, Dr. Thomas A. Outland, Howard E. Bishop, and Dr. Rodney L. Stedge; (fourth row) Dr. John W. Bradley, Dr. Daniel J. Gary, Dr. Howard K. Gray, Dr. R. Wallace Teed, Dr. Lester S. Knapp, and Dr. William Bache.

Five

The 1930s Are a Decade of Change

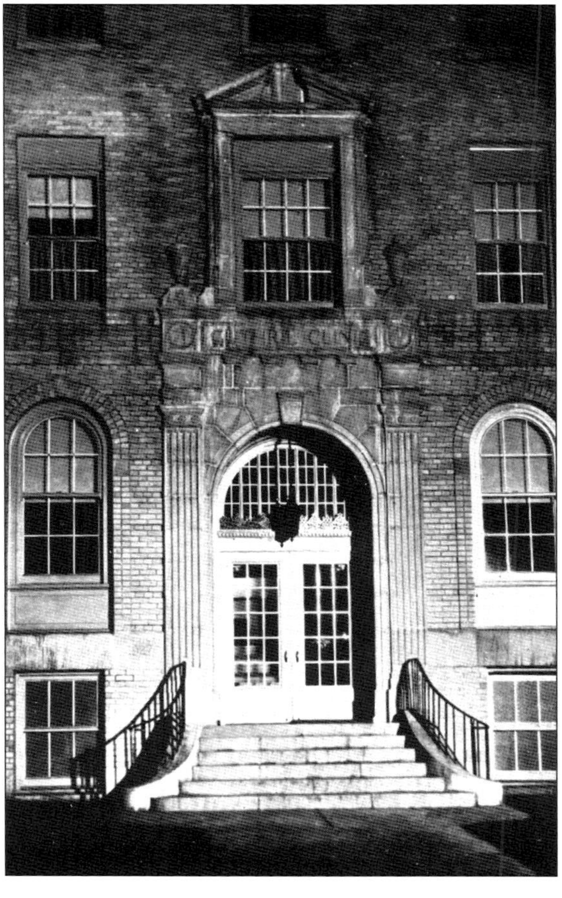

The new entrance to the Guthrie Clinic building added to the prestige of the clinic and Robert Packer Hospital. These steps still exist and lead from the lobby of the Bird Sumner Building to the third floor of the hospital.

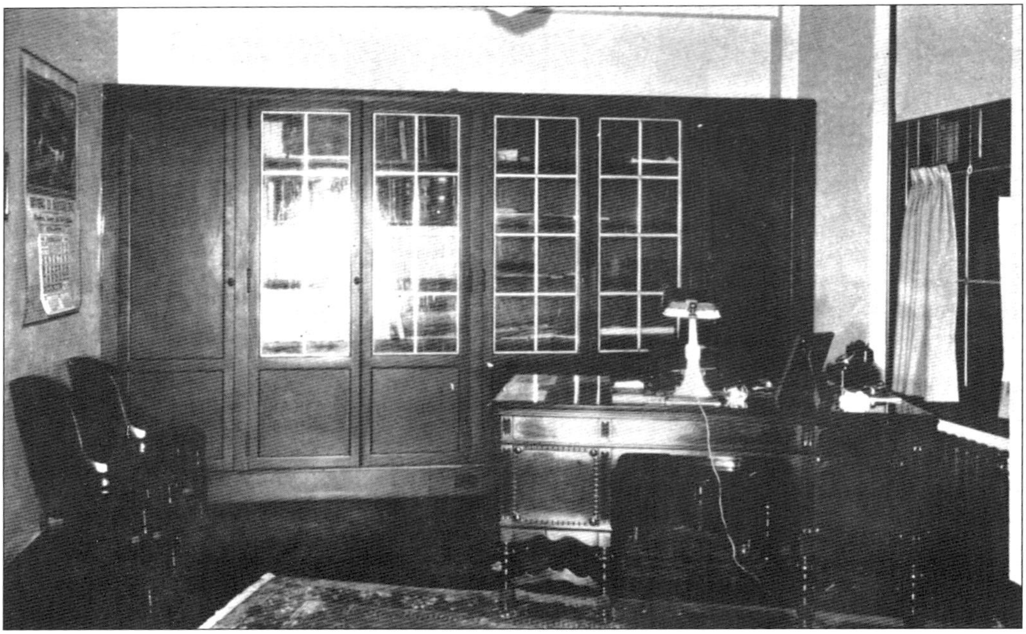
The Guthrie Clinic building constructed in 1928 housed the superintendent's office, shown here in 1930.

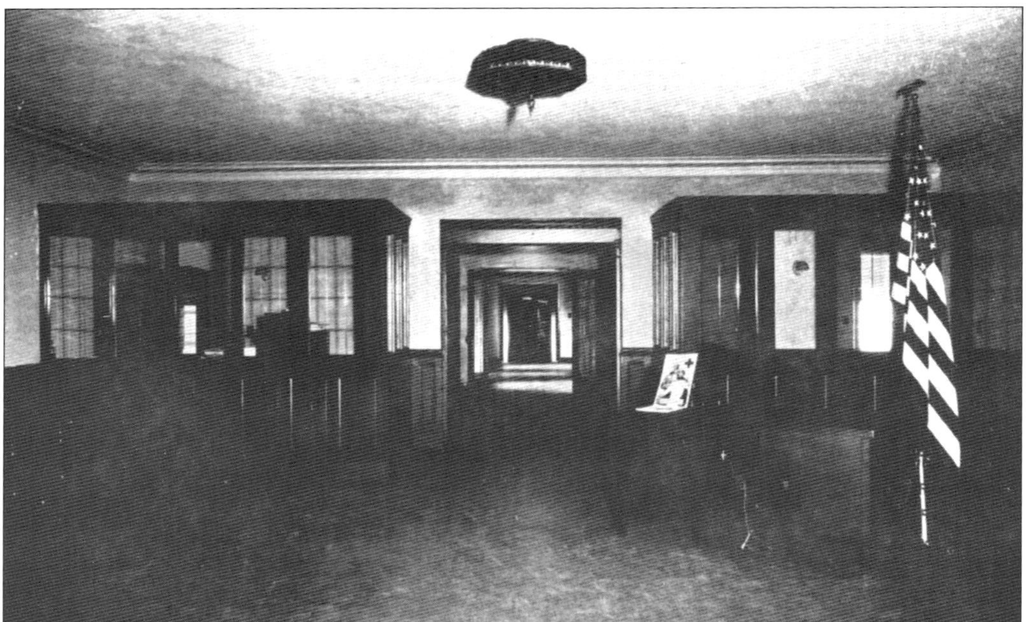
The Guthrie Clinic lobby (pictured here in 1930) still exists today on the third floor of the hospital, just outside the office of the president and chief executive officer of Guthrie Healthcare System.

The Guthrie Clinic building contained space for the dental department, shown here with updated dental equipment in 1930.

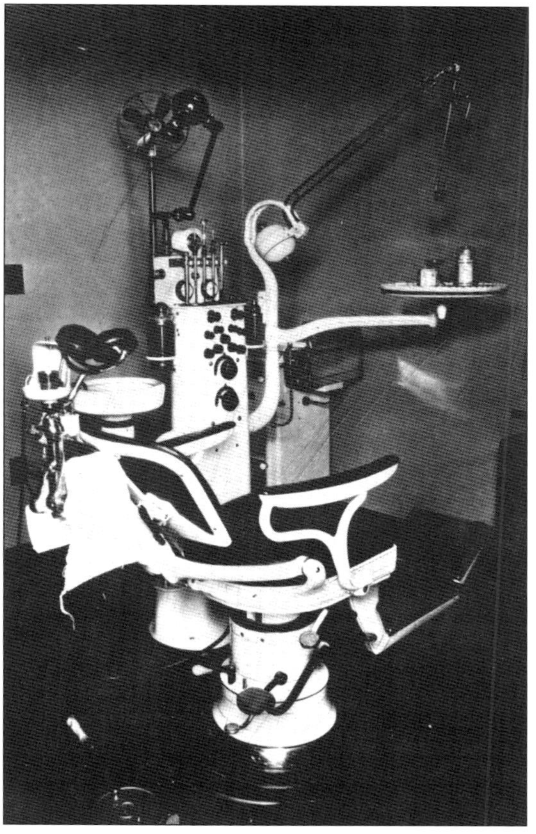

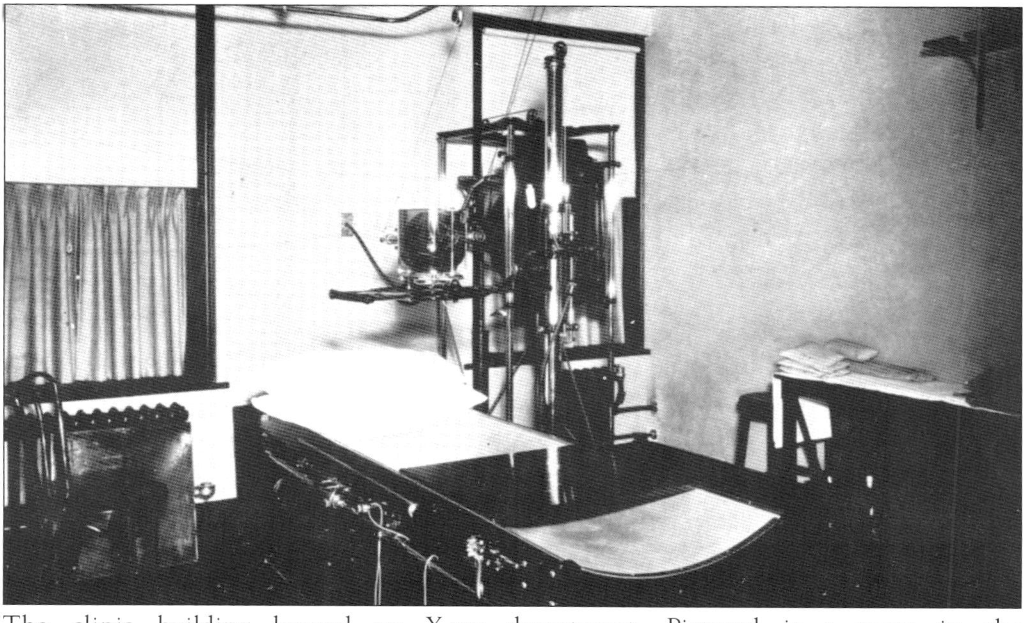

The clinic building housed an X-ray department. Pictured is a room in the department around 1930.

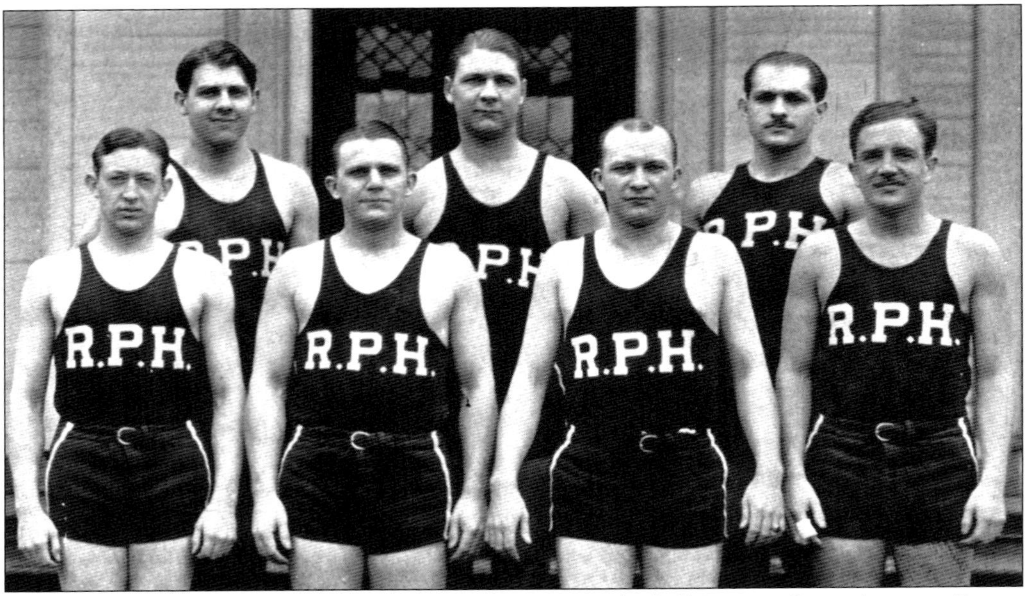

These physicians were the champions of the Keystone Basketball League, Sayre Amateur Sports Association. Members of the interns champion team from 1931 to 1932 are, from left to right, (first row) Dr. William Copenhaver, Dr. Raymond Evans, Dr. Steven Collins, and Dr. Harvey Klaer Jr.; (second row) Dr. William C. Beck, Dr. Charles Yarrington, and Dr. Irvin Ershler.

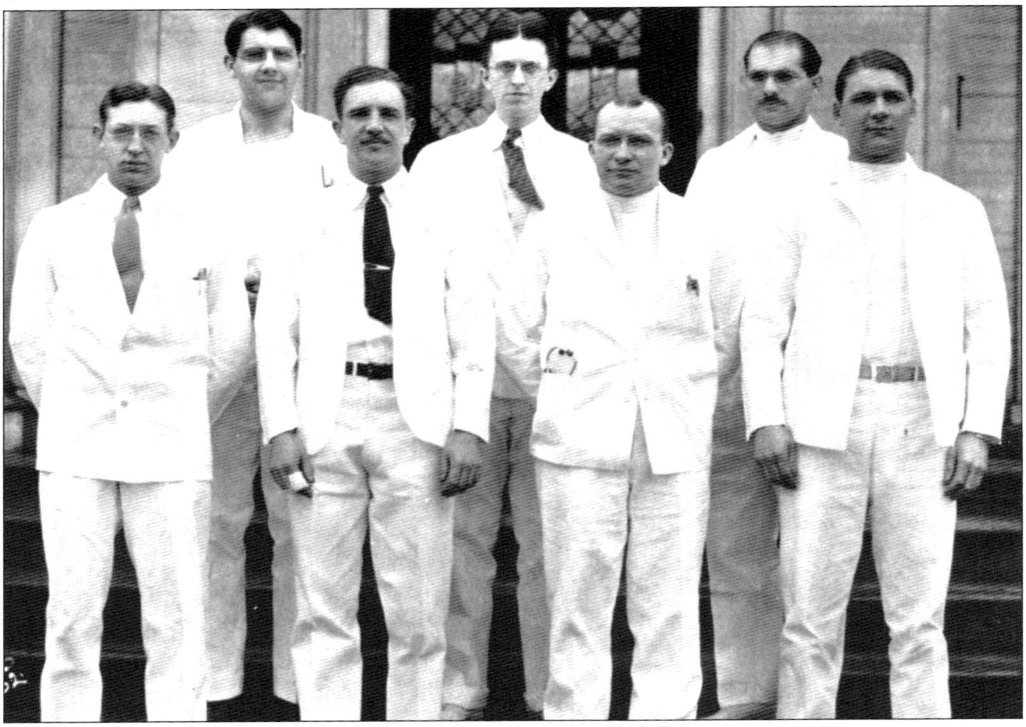

Hospital interns from 1932 include, from left to right, (first row) Dr. William Copenhaver, Dr. Harvey Klaer Jr., Dr. Steven Collins, and Dr. Charles Yarrington; (second row) Dr. William C. Beck, Dr. Clifton Lynch, and Dr. Irvin Ershler.

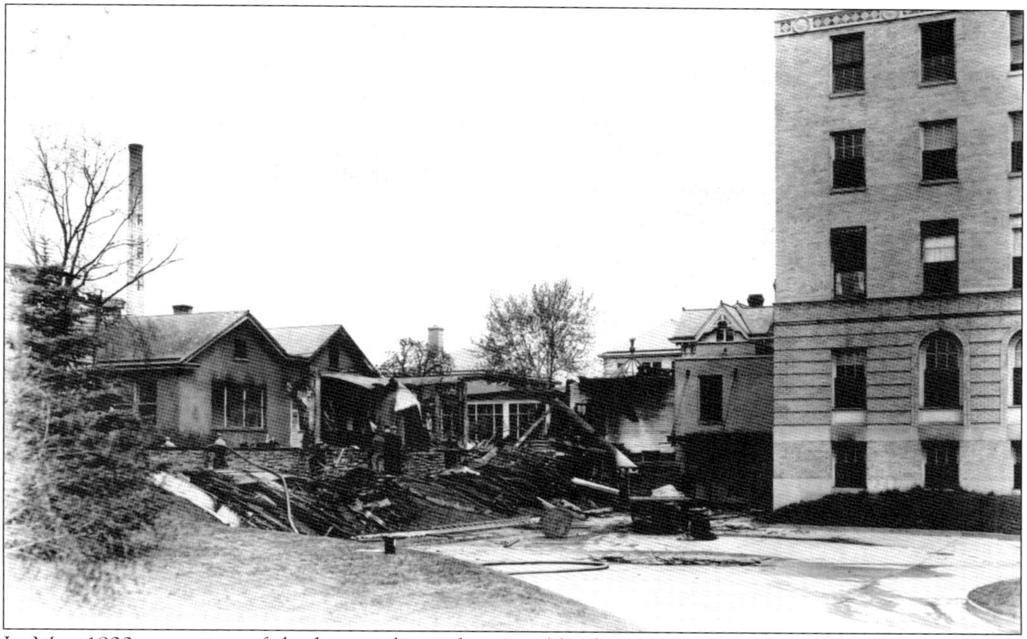

In May 1933, a section of the hospital was destroyed by fire. It was one of the most disheartening times in Dr. Donald Guthrie's life. But within 48 hours after the catastrophe, patient care resumed and steps were taken to erect a new hospital. The building still standing on the right was the Guthrie Clinic building, which is now the Bird Sumner Building.

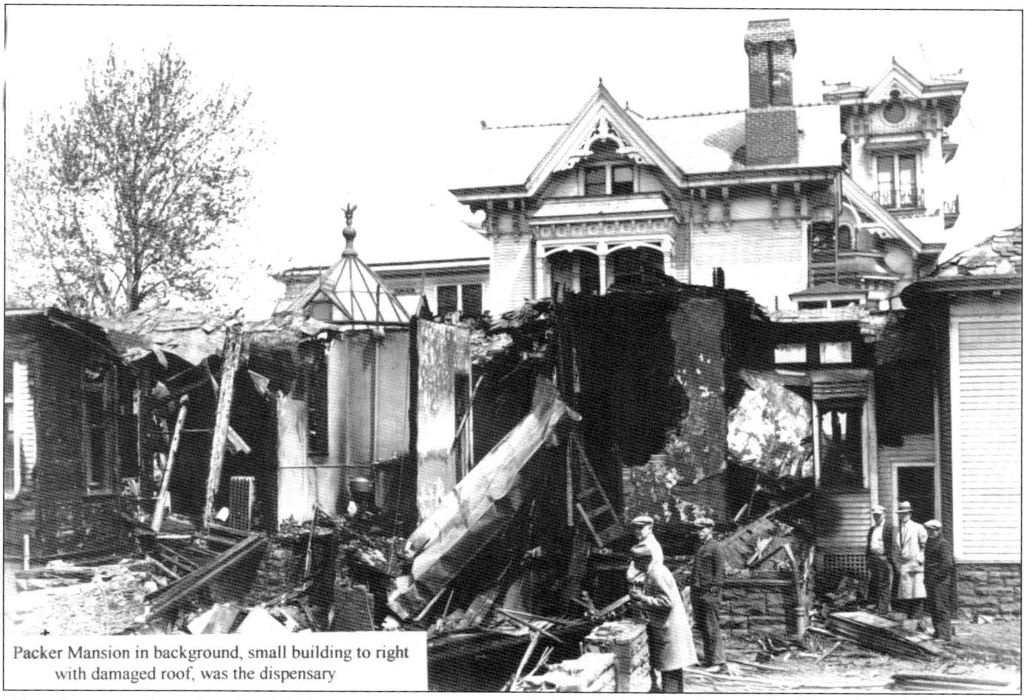
Packer Mansion in background, small building to right
with damaged roof, was the dispensary

The damage done by the 1933 fire was in excess of $500,000. In this photograph, Packer Mansion is visible behind the burned building.

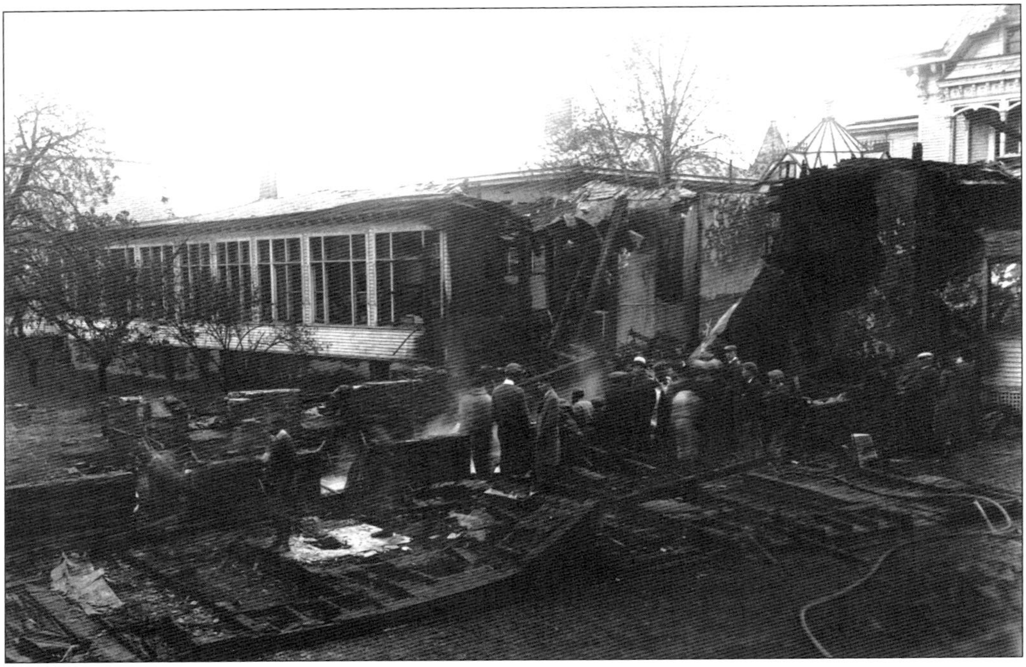

This is another view of the damage done by the fire, which was discovered in a basement storeroom.

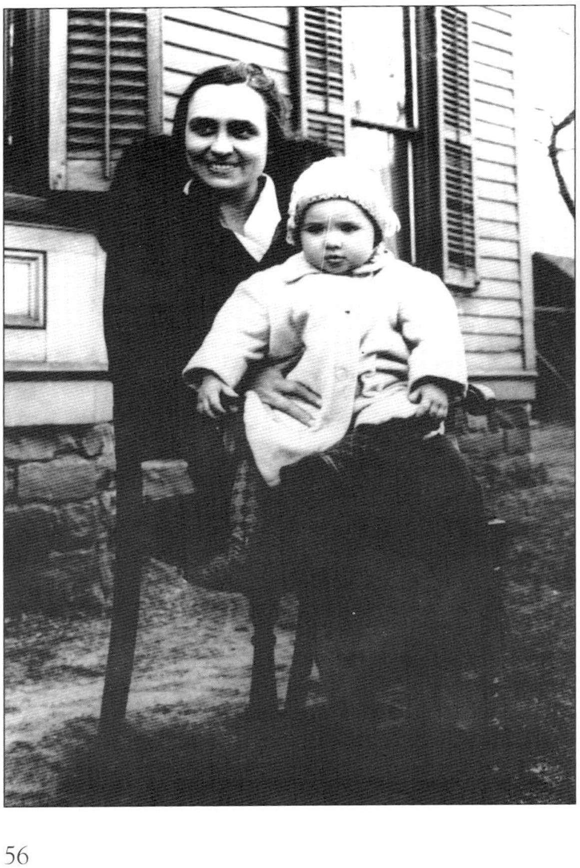

Patients were evacuated when the fire broke out, but Dr. John Higgins and Dr. David Taylor worked by flashlight to deliver a baby girl to Ray and Reta Lewis of Chemung Street in Sayre. Immediately after the baby's birth, a fireman carried her to the Coleman Memorial Parish House next door. Reta was carried in a bed to her home. Pictured are Reta Lewis and her daughter Roslyn.

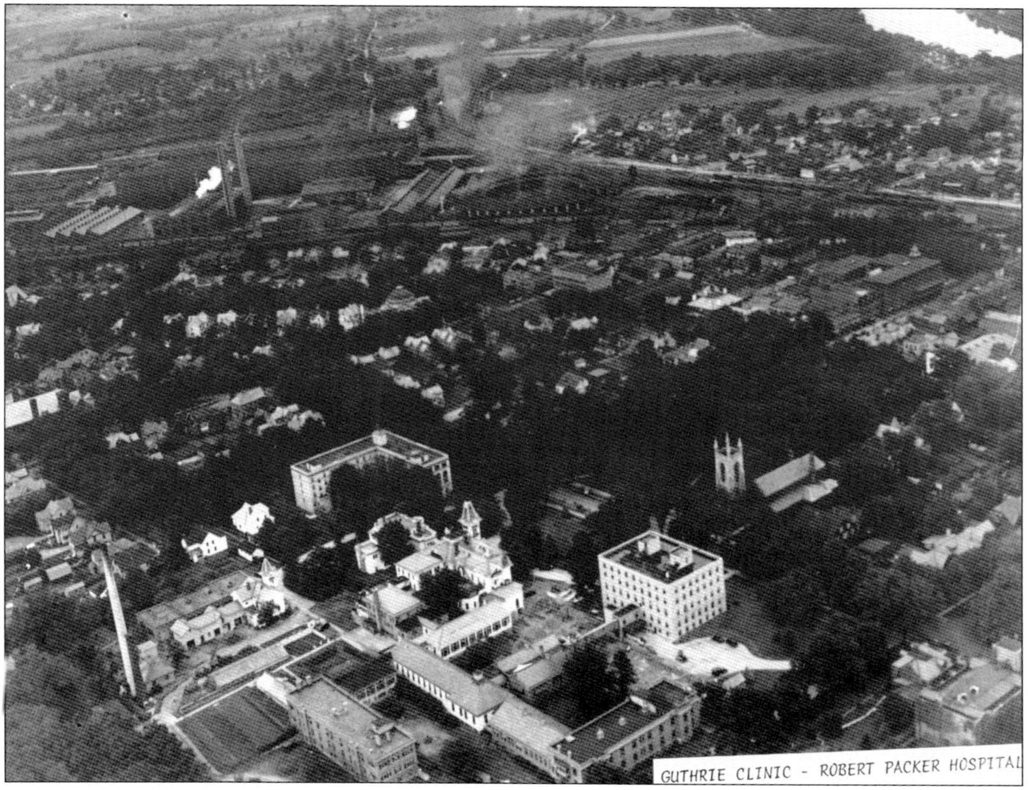

The damage done by the fire is visible in this aerial view of the campus of Robert Packer Hospital and Guthrie Clinic in 1933.

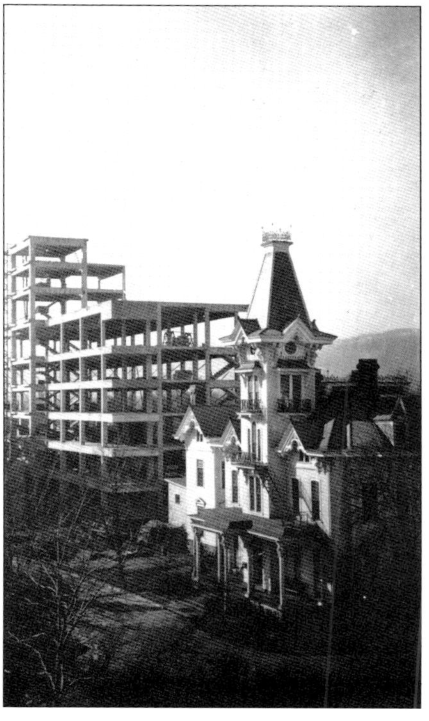

The afternoon after the fire, the board of trustees voted to start construction of a new $300,000 facility to be built from plans that had been on the drawing board since 1929. The seven-story structure would raise the hospital's bed capacity to 285. Shown here is the steel framing of the new facility, next to Packer Mansion.

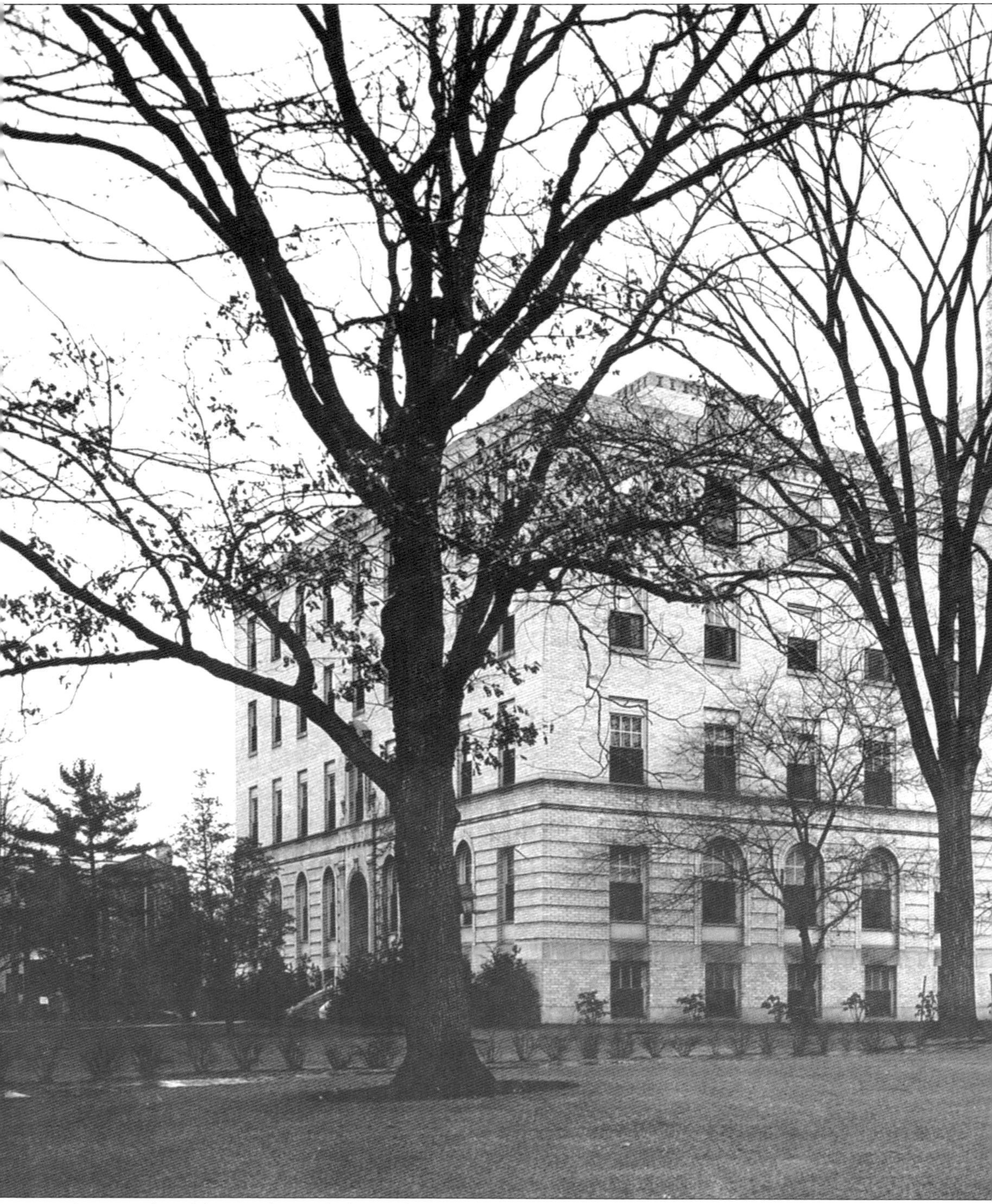

The completed hospital was dedicated on December 6, 1934. The money received from the fire insurance—$98,875—did not cover the cost of the new building, and the board decided not to hold a fund-raising drive. After months of trying to procure funds, the hospital received a

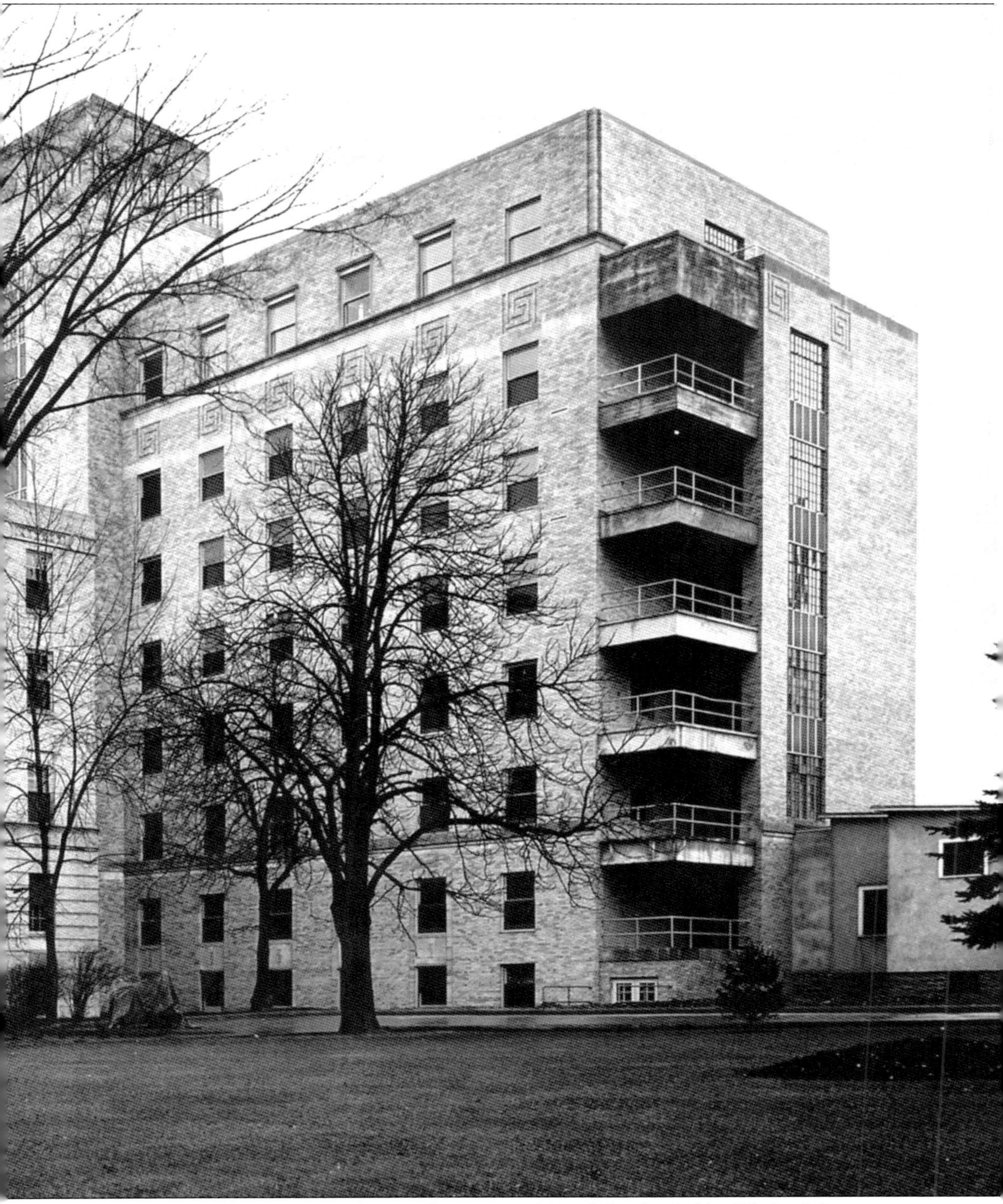

contract for the purchase of Robert Packer Hospital Bonds by the Public Works Administration supporting a federal loan of up to $420,000. The Guthrie Clinic is in the foreground.

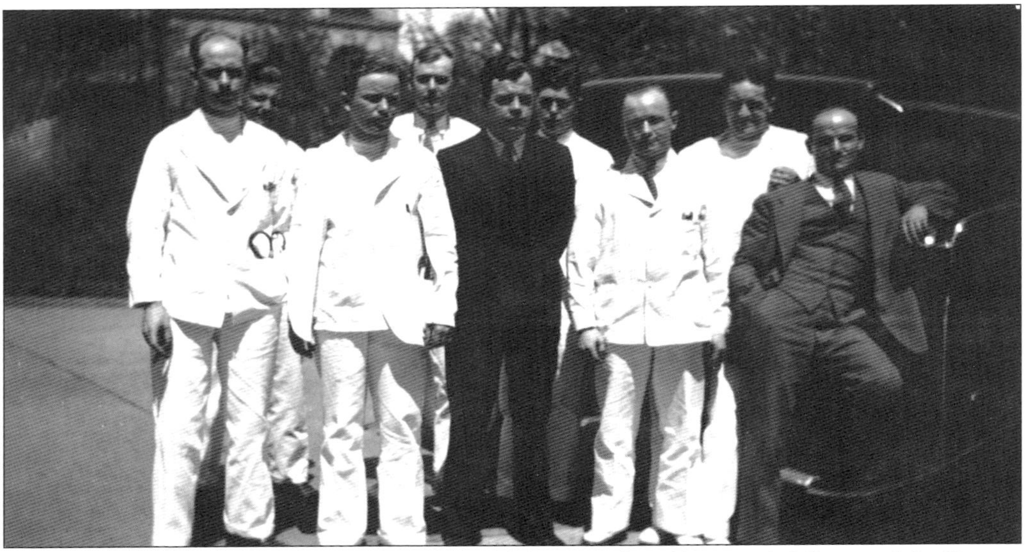
Hospital interns in March 1933 are, from left to right, (first row) Thomas MacGregor, Henry McGuire, ? Gillen, Wilfred Langly, and Thomas Dimitroff; (second row) David Taylor, James Appel, Parker Horton, and James Reddington.

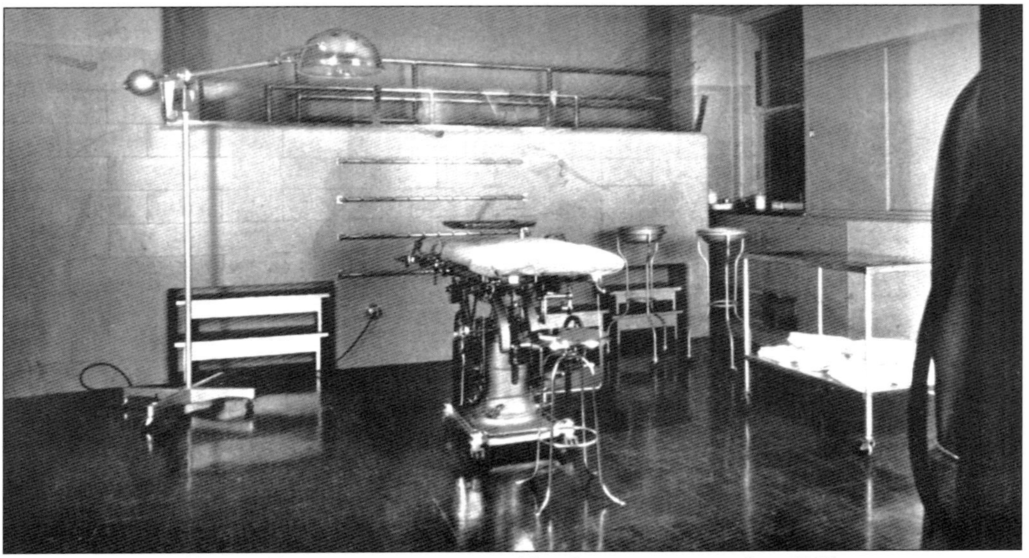
The new hospital housed large operating rooms like this one, pictured in 1935.

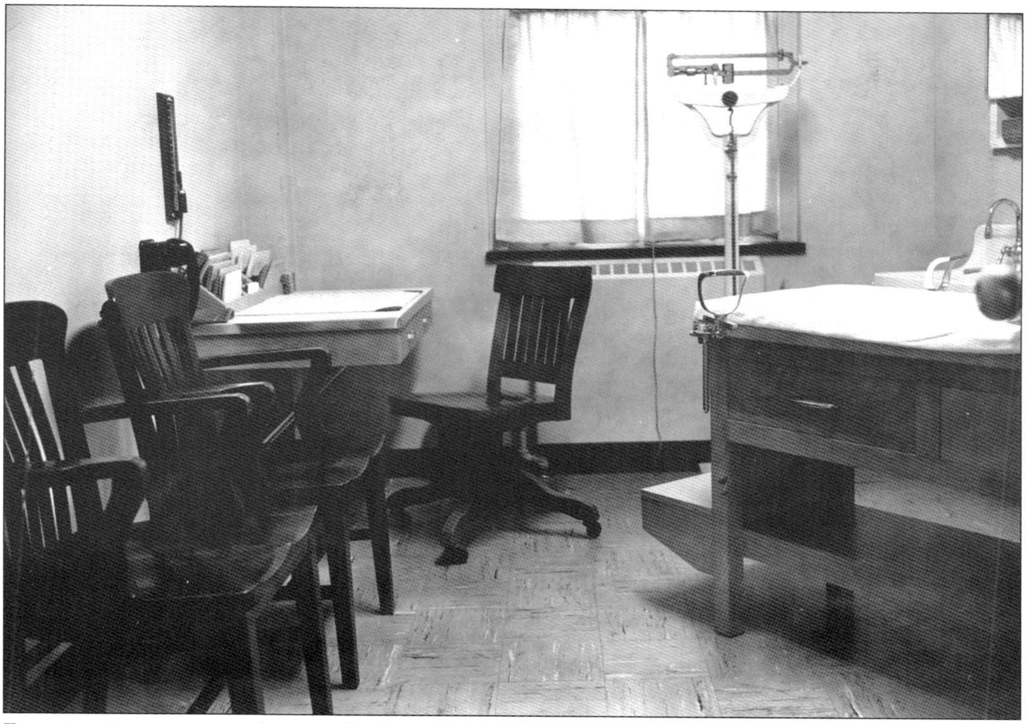

Examination rooms in the new facility were modern and spacious.

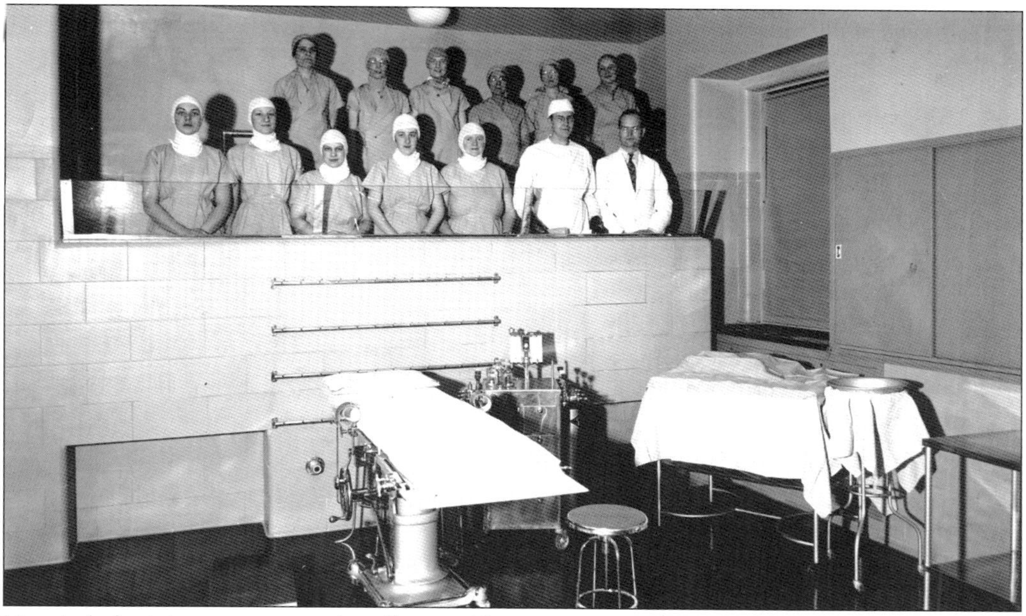

Hospital physicians, nurses, and staff were able to view procedures in the operating room of the new hospital. Assembled in the operating room are, from left to right, (first row) Clare Jacobs, Edna Anthony, Winnie Jones, unidentified, Lil Kerhler, Bill Fowler, and Dr. Willis Redding; (second row) Belle Foote, Violette Brooks, Ann Wildrick, Lora Scott, Dorothy Fishler, and Eleanor Drislane.

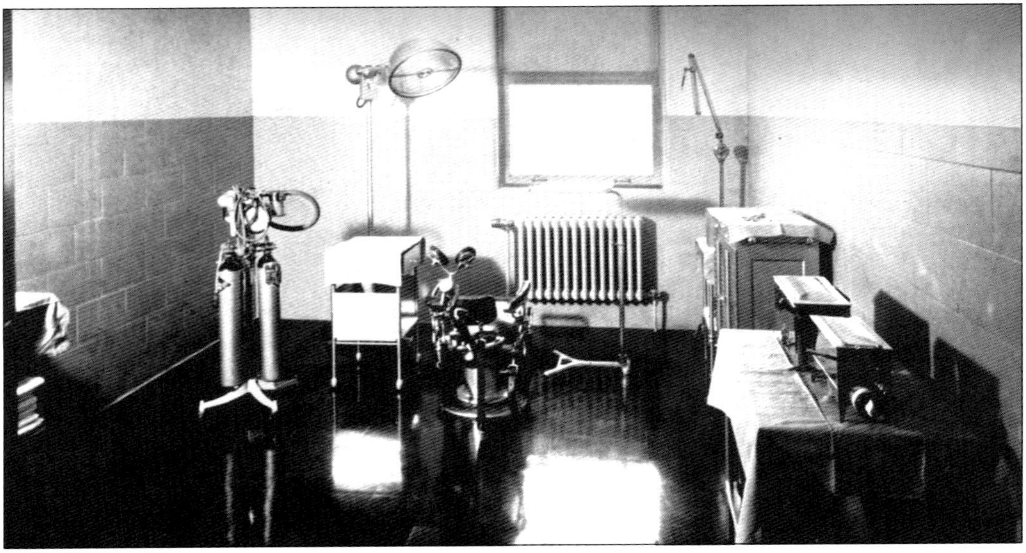

The new hospital had an operating room dedicated to dental procedures.

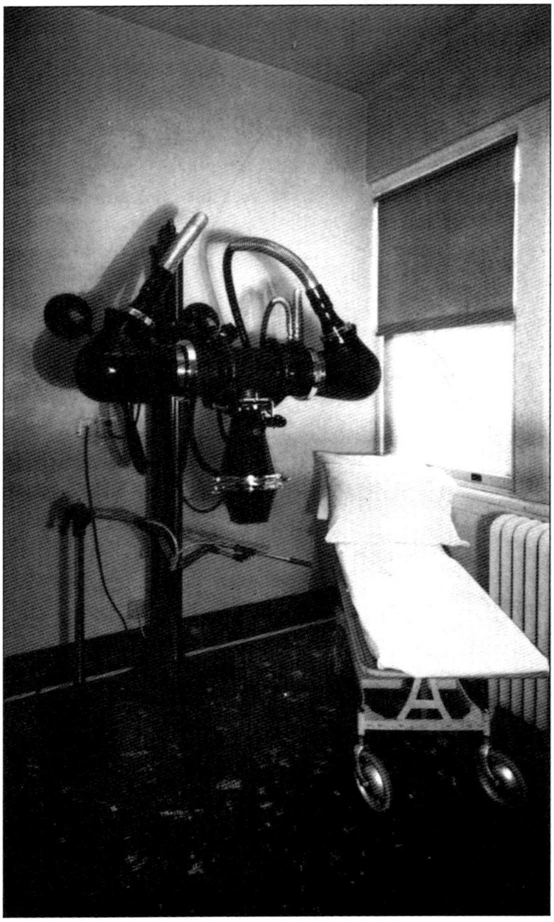

A deep therapy room was also a part of the new hospital.

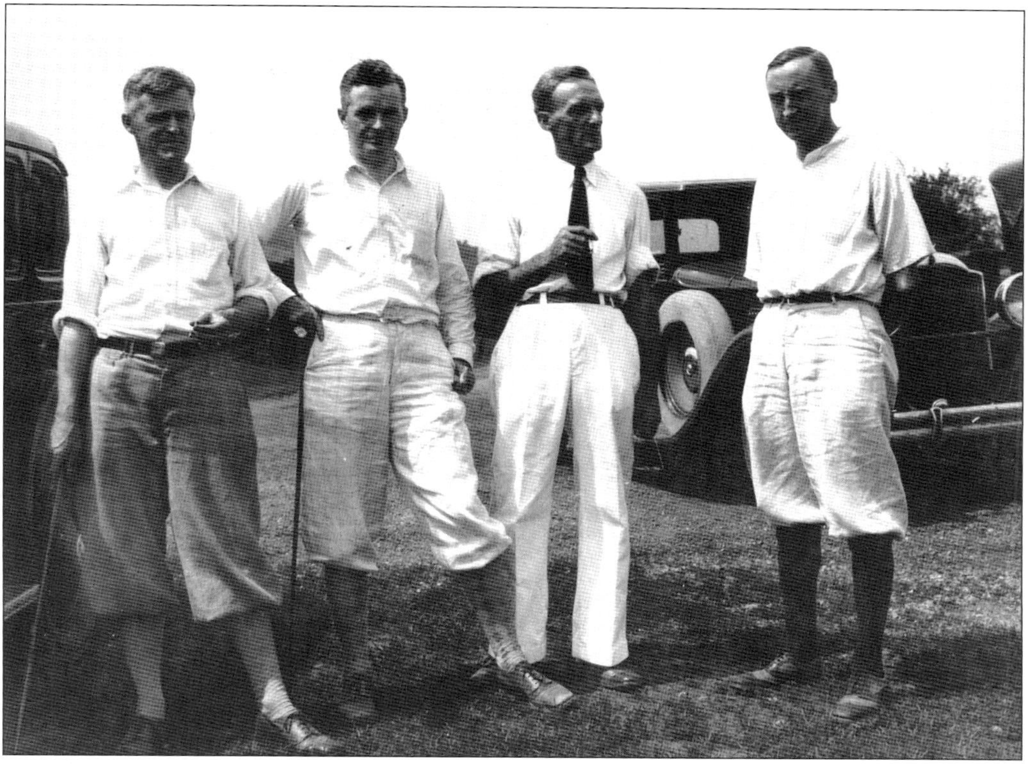

From left to right, hospital staff Ira Kurtz, Red Roach, X-ray operator Sydney T. Purkiss, and Dr. Charles A. DeWan enjoy a golf outing.

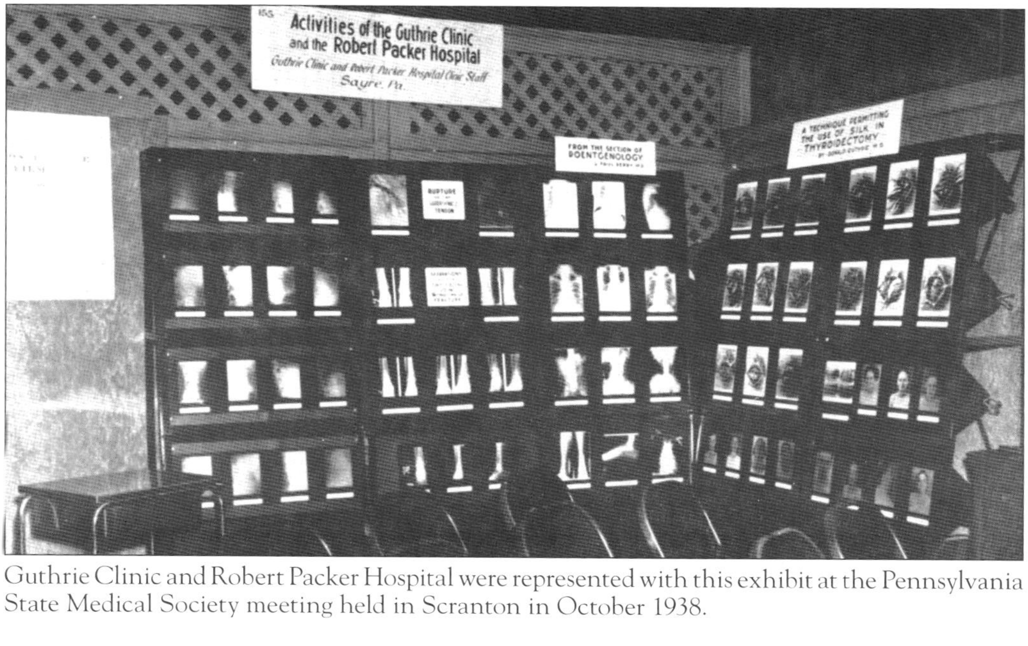

Guthrie Clinic and Robert Packer Hospital were represented with this exhibit at the Pennsylvania State Medical Society meeting held in Scranton in October 1938.

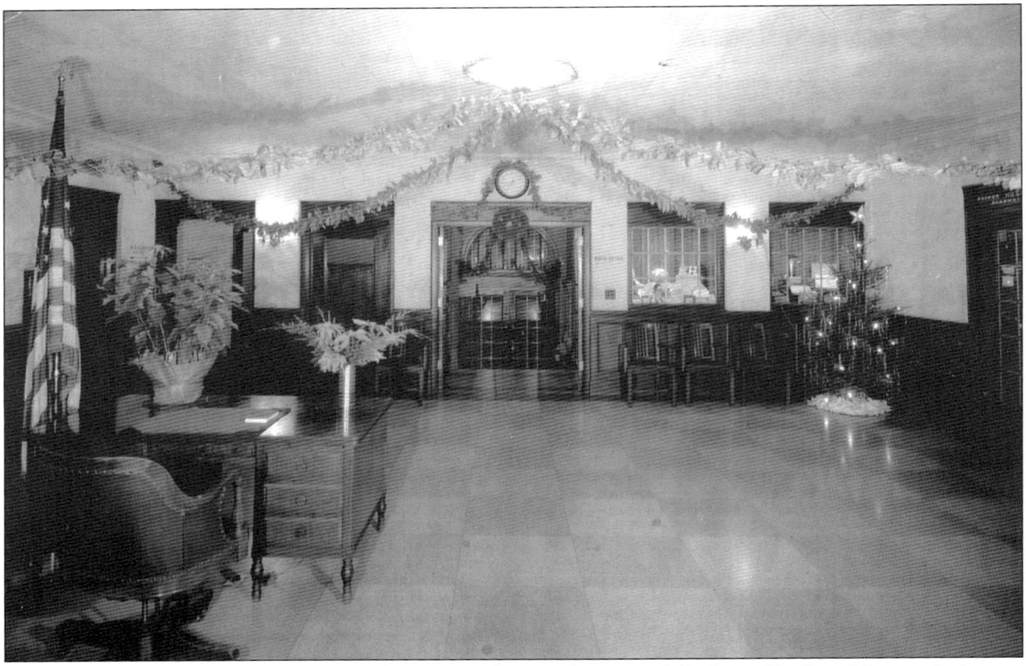

Festive decorations adorn the lobby of Guthrie Clinic and Robert Packer Hospital during the holiday season.

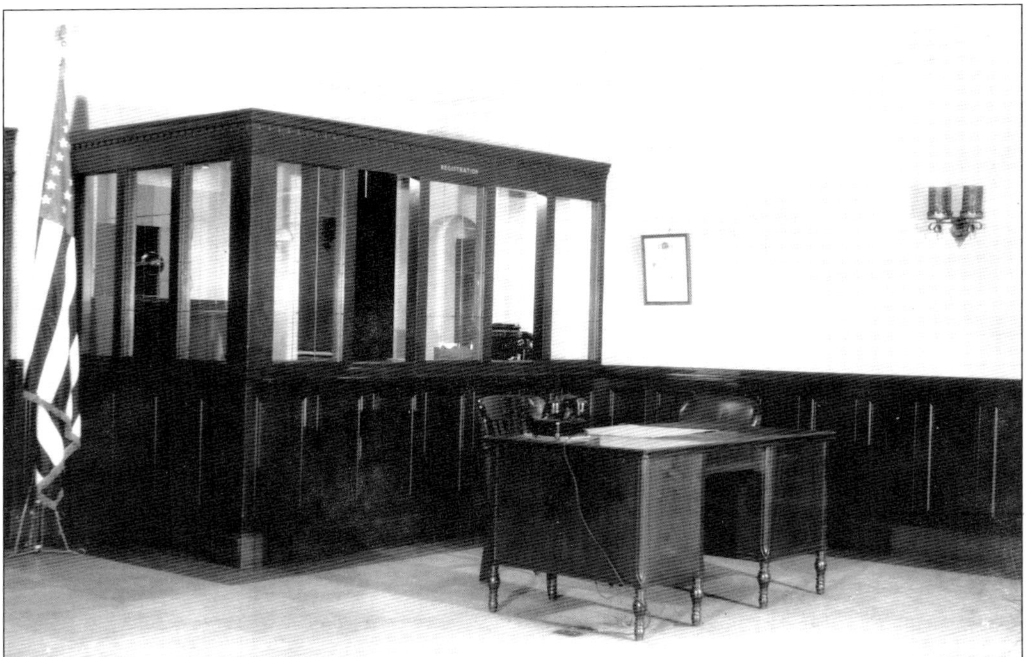

The telephone exchange and registration desk in Guthrie Clinic were located in the lobby.

Six

Guthrie's Reputation Grows

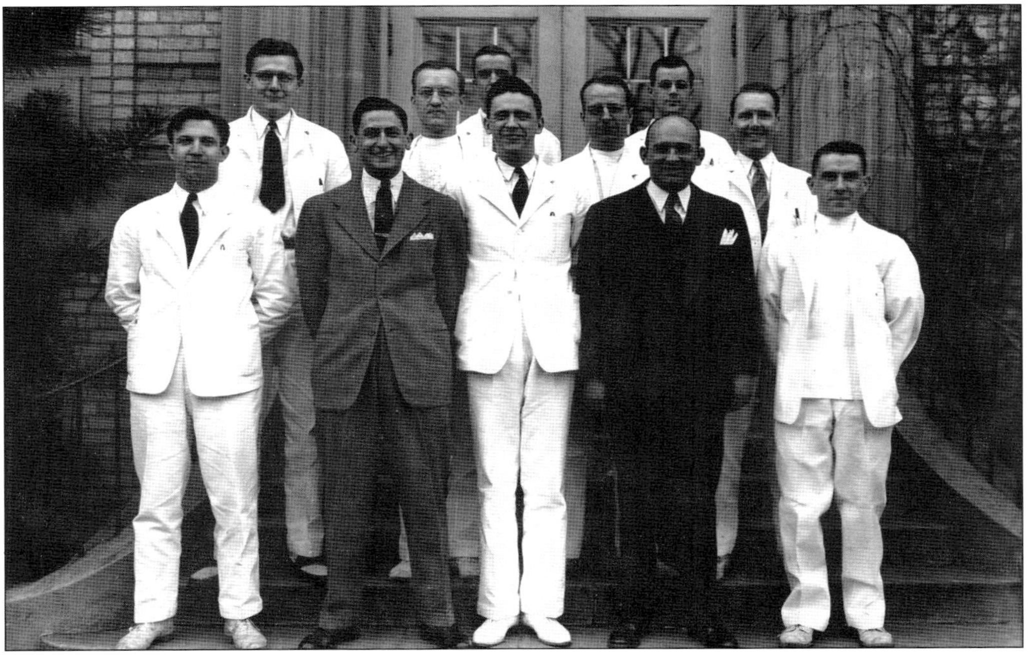

In 1942, the following served as hospital interns and fellows, from left to right, (first row) Drs. F. O'Brien, I. Schimmel, W. Jacobs, P. Shank, and O. Gordon; (second row) Drs. K. Rague, S. Buckley, A. Butler, and W. Cavallano; (third row) Drs. G. Hanlon and E. Newhart.

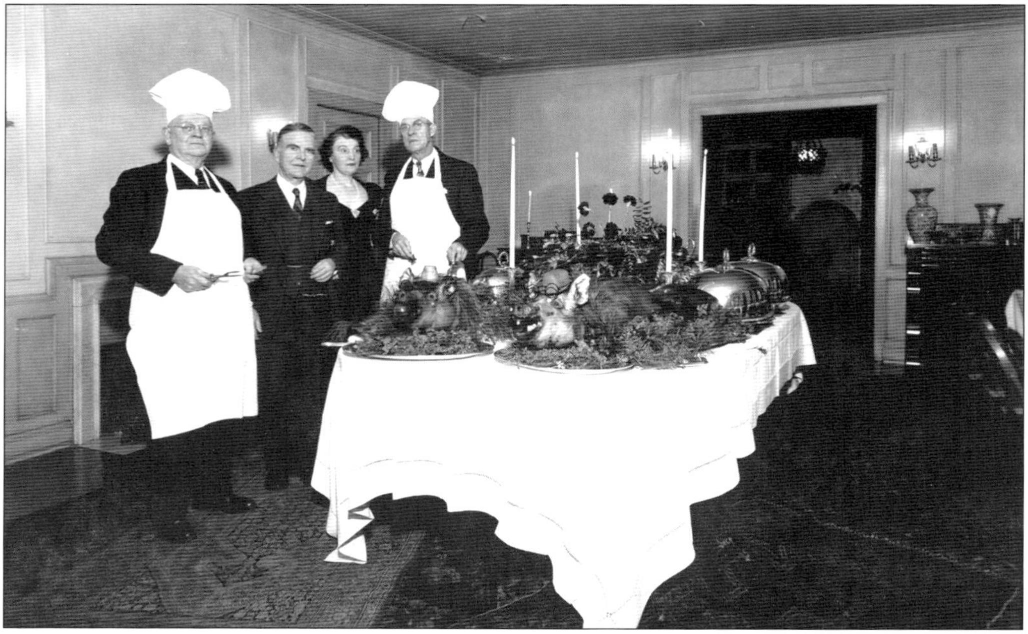

Dr. Donald and Emily Baker Guthrie hosted an annual pig dinner at their home for clinic physicians, local doctors, and close friends. Emily was the only woman included in the festivities. The menu consisted of roast pig, sauerkraut, creamed onions, mashed potatoes, vanilla ice cream, and a special, superb chocolate sauce. In this photograph, from left to right, Dr. George W. Hawk, Dr. Donald Guthrie, Emily Baker Guthrie, and Dr. George F. Carling are ready to start carving.

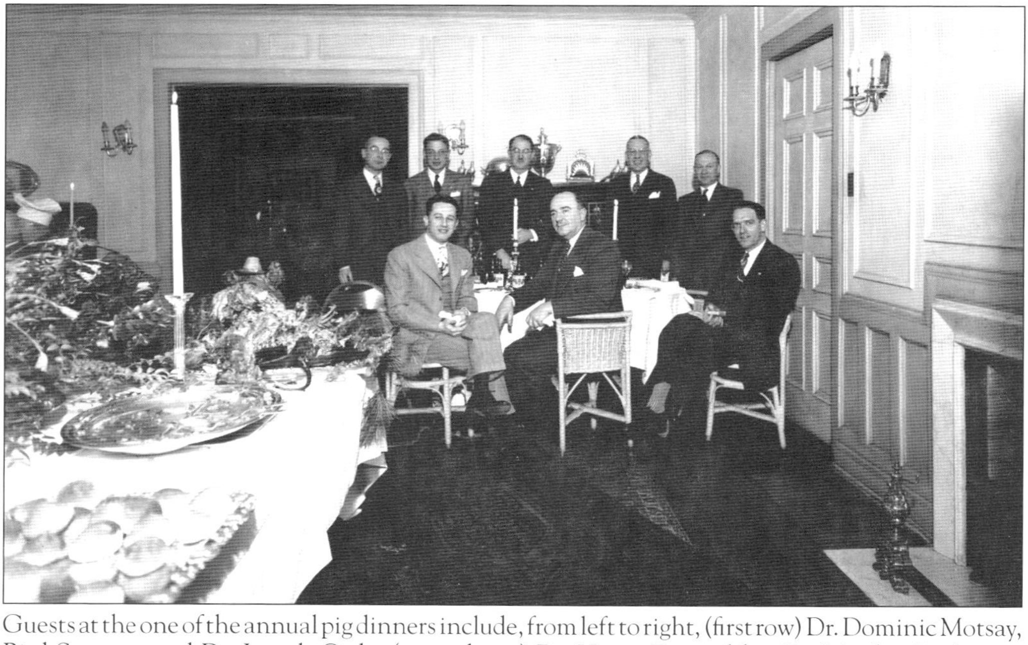

Guests at the one of the annual pig dinners include, from left to right, (first row) Dr. Dominic Motsay, Bird Sumner, and Dr. Joseph Cady; (second row) Dr. Henry Rentschler, Dr. Manley Rockman, Dr. Paul Perry, unidentified, and Dr. Stanley D. Conklin.

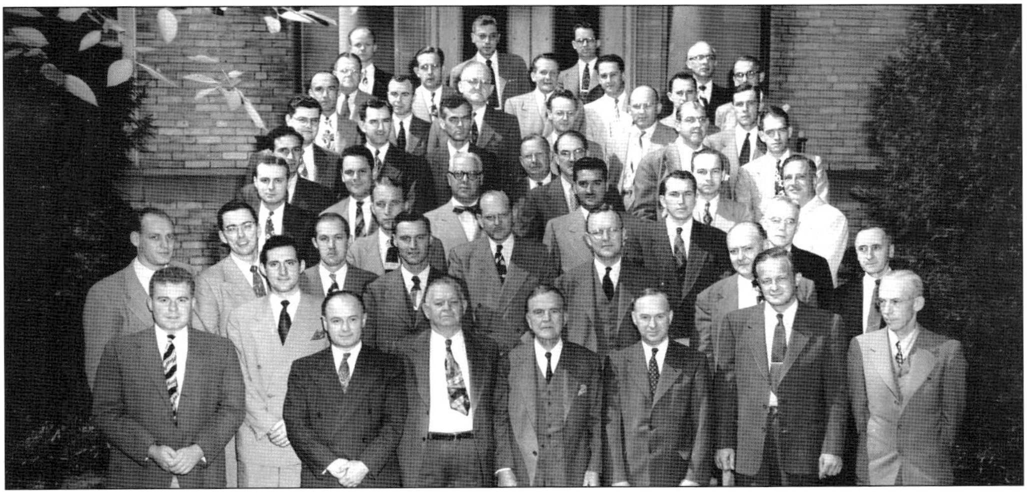

In September 1949, the annual meeting of the Association of Residents and Former Residents of Guthrie Clinic and Robert Packer Hospital drew quite a crowd. Dr. Guthrie is in the center of the first row. Pictured are (in no particular order) William Dotter, John Bryfogle, W. D. Langley, George W. Hawk, Donald Guthrie, Stanley D. Conklin, George Harnwood, unidentified, Elting C. Johnson, Joseph Hemming, Fred Rook, unidentified, William F. Brehm, unidentified, Paul Shallenberger, John Higgins, Charles DeWan, Philip Frey, Robert Kerr, Harry Armitage, Hugh Robertson, Gerald Gagnon, Wayne Allen, Donald Clough, Harvey Klaer Jr., Jean Brochu, unidentified, Paul Perry, John Delaney, James Flood, Axel Olsen, Jesse Littleton, Irvin Eishler, William C. Beck, unidentified, Joseph Cady, ? Helm, unidentified, William Bourys, ? Kornegy, Dominic Motsay, Gene Komiski, Henry D. Rentschler, Frederick Sanford, Ralph Matson, Don Baker, Manley Rockman, Ronald Prindle, and Malin Martin.

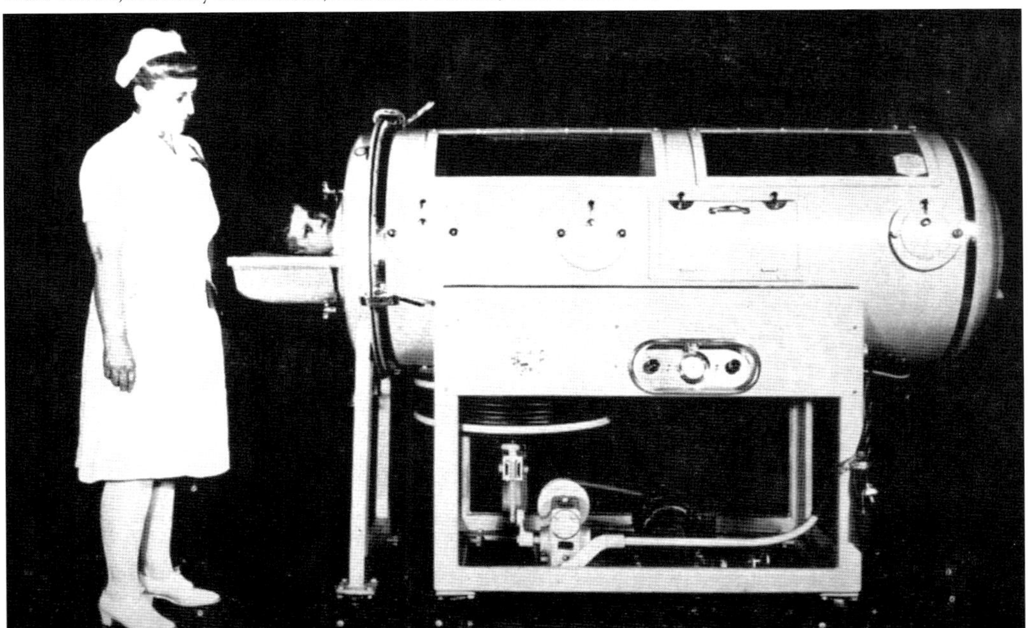

Patients with polio were treated with the Drinker-Collins respirator, an iron lung, shown here with Bernice Bertelsen, RN, around 1942.

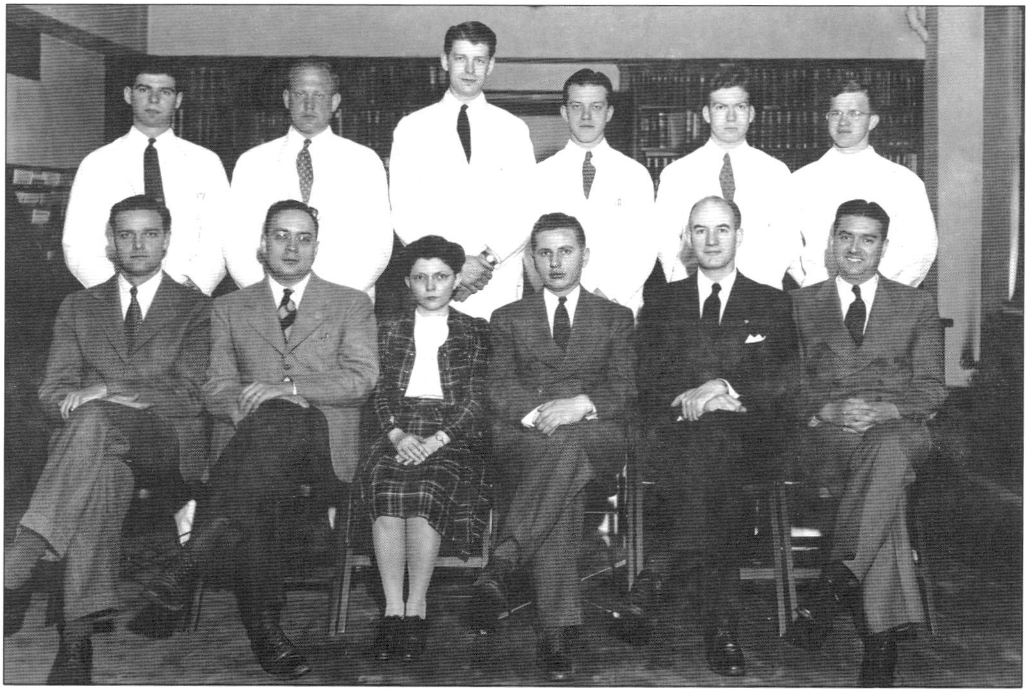

In 1945, the following served as hospital fellows and interns, from left to right, (first row) Drs. Virgil May, T. Toland, Betty Suess, John Suess, P. Hardin, and Gerald Gagon; (second row) Drs. Samuel Meltzer, Thomas B. Johnson, Stanley Moore, James McVay, Don King, and Joseph Wilson.

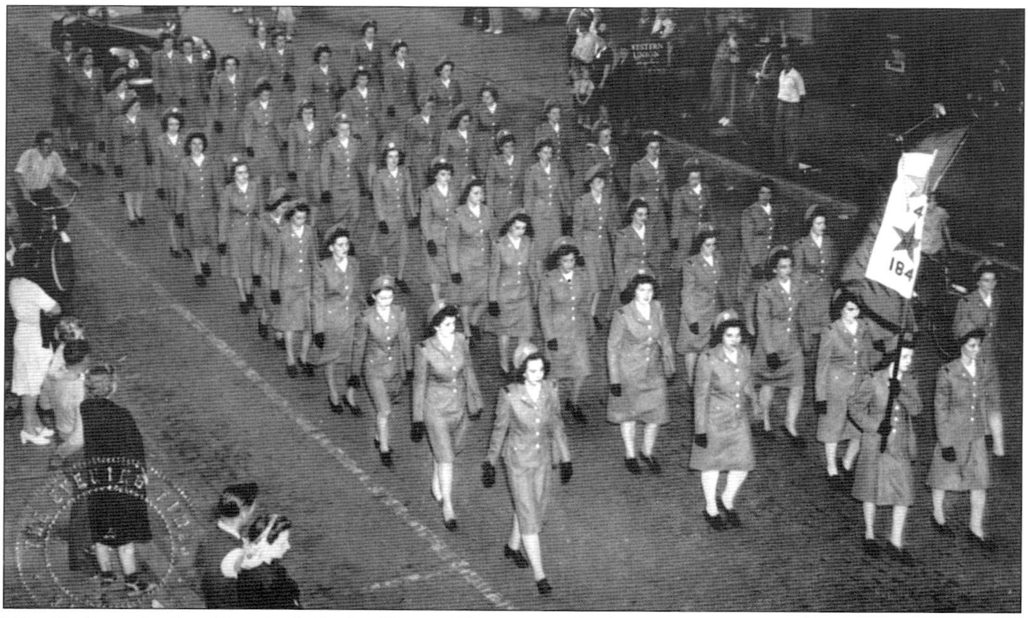

The Robert Packer Hospital Cadet Nurse Corps marched in a victory parade in 1945.

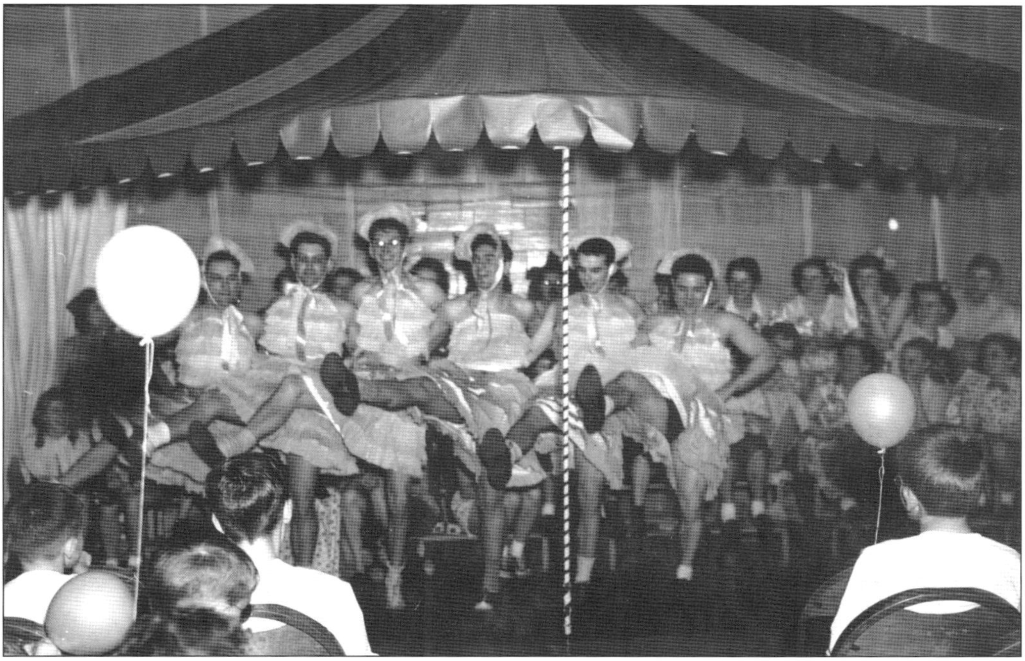

One of the most talked about events in the history of the organization was the annual circus, first held in 1947. Here six versatile Robert Packer Hospital interns perform as the Rockettes. Pictured are, from left to right, Drs. Richard Markee, Jose Quijano, ? Smythe, John Watson, Arthur Coddington, and Robert Delaplaine.

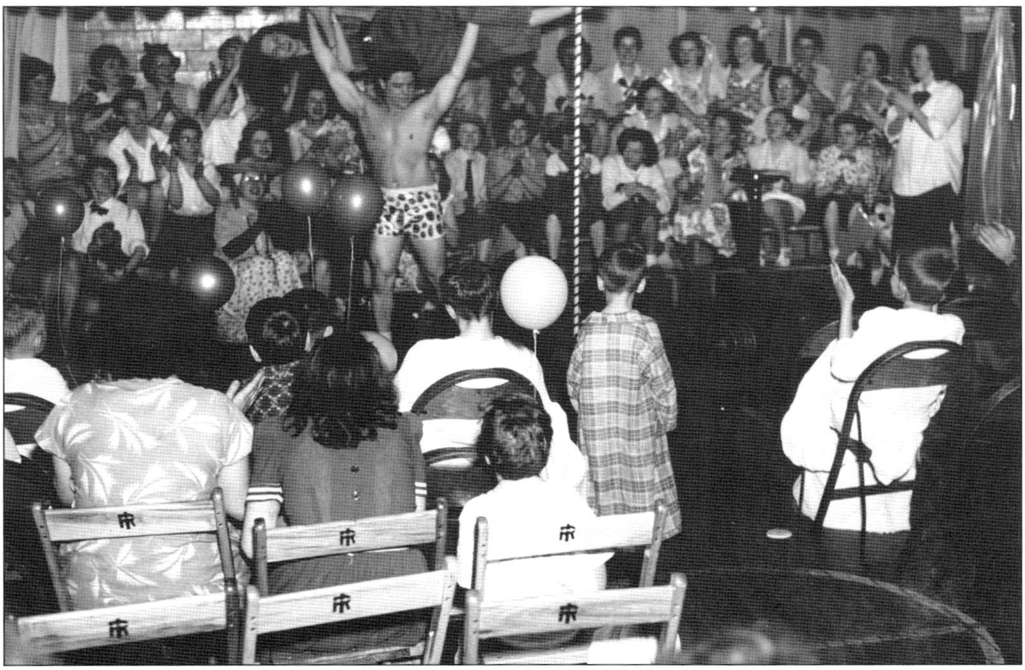

Dr. Robert Delaplaine entertains the little patients from the children's ward at a preview of the circus.

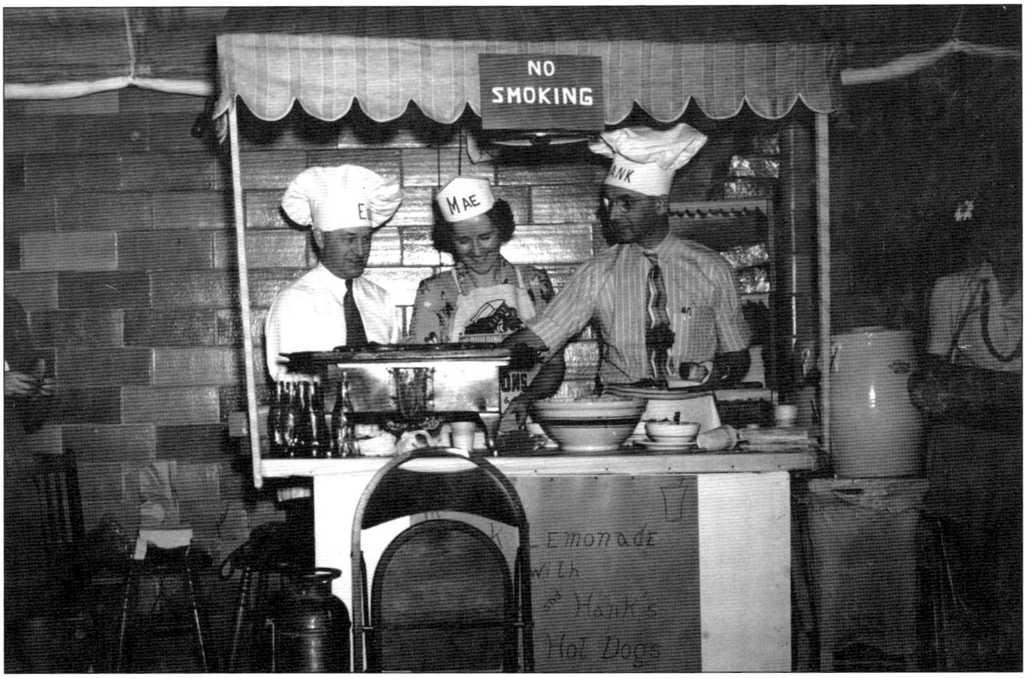

In this view of the activities at the circus, "Ed," "Mae," and "Hank" served up refreshments. Running the concession stand are, from left to right, Dr. Stanley D. Conklin; Florence E. Miller, RN; and Dr. Henry D. Rentschler.

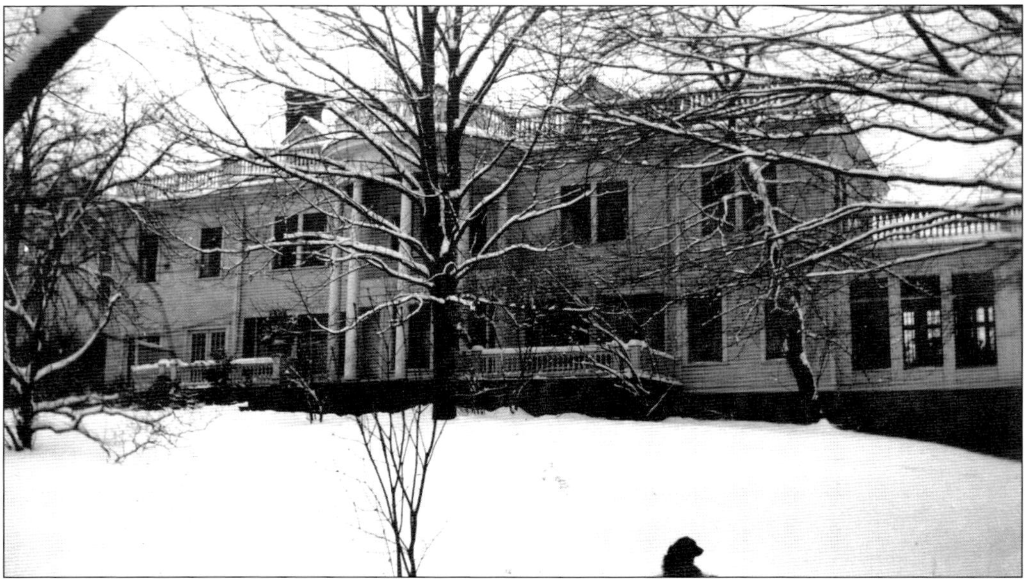

This photograph of the Guthries' residence was used on a personal Christmas card from Dr. Donald and Emily Baker Guthrie. The home was provided to the surgeon in chief and was extensively renovated and enlarged in 1919.

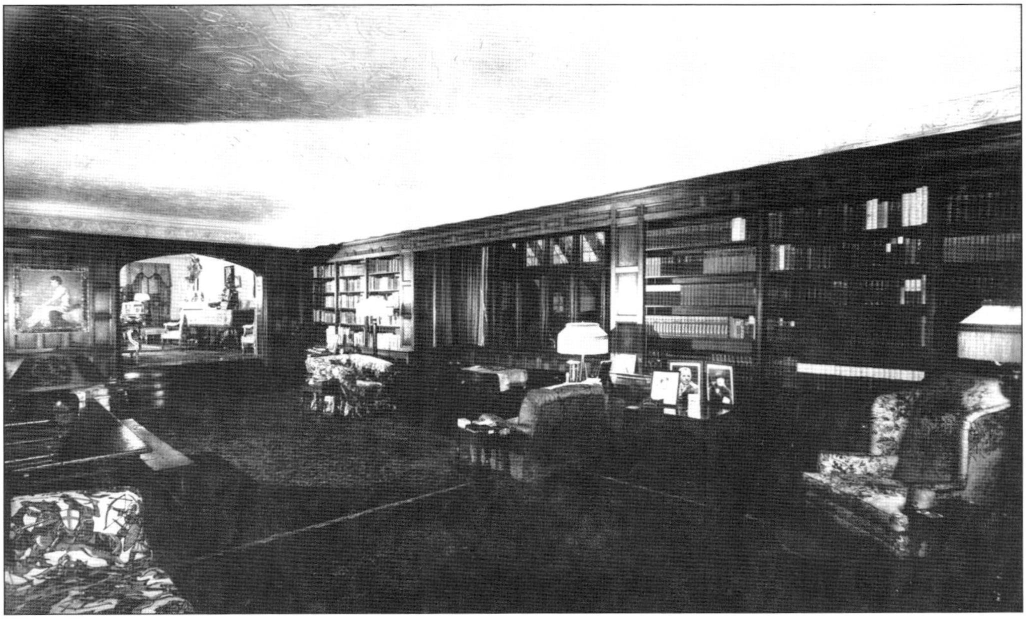

This photograph shows the Guthries' home after the renovation.

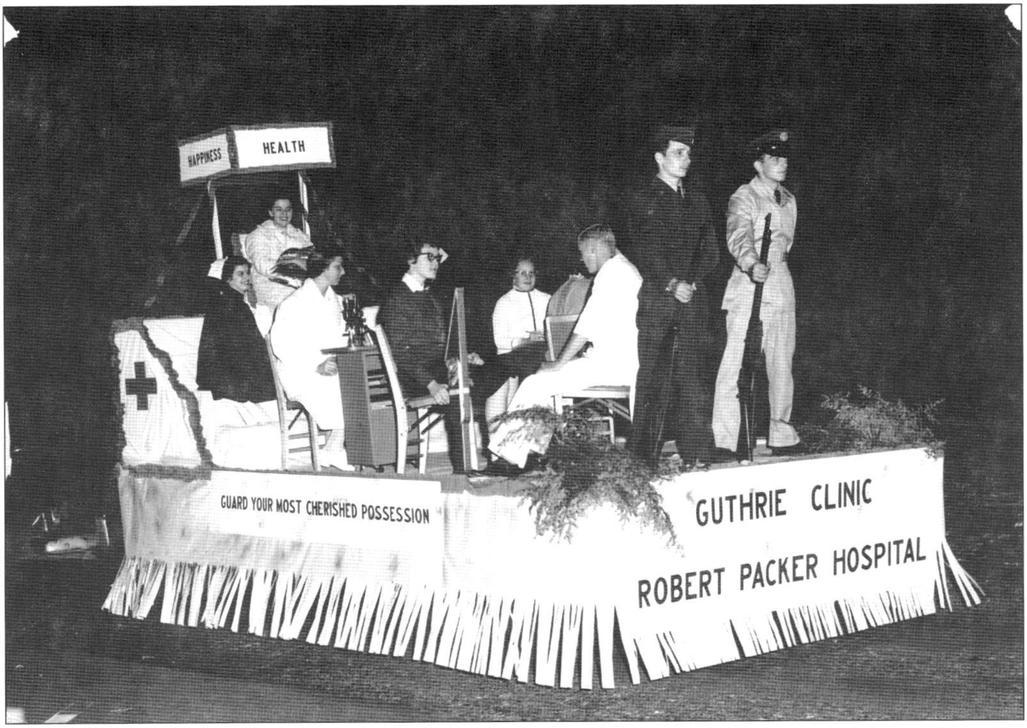

Guthrie Clinic and Robert Packer Hospital staff participate in a Halloween parade.

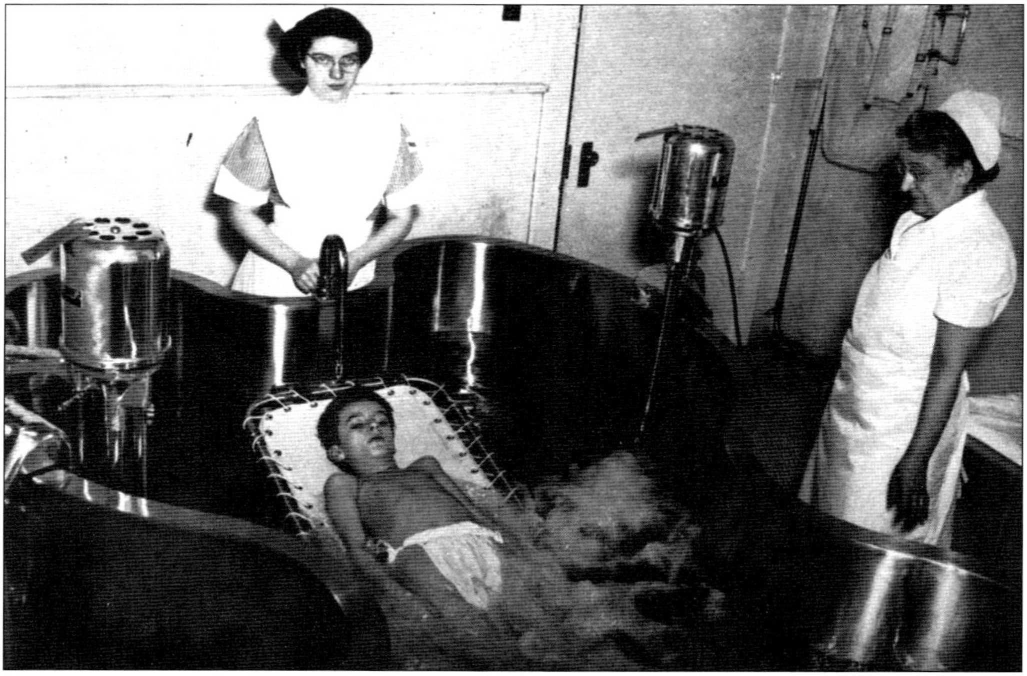

Continuing to employ the latest technologies, the Hubbard tank was used for patients who might benefit from warm-water hydrotherapy.

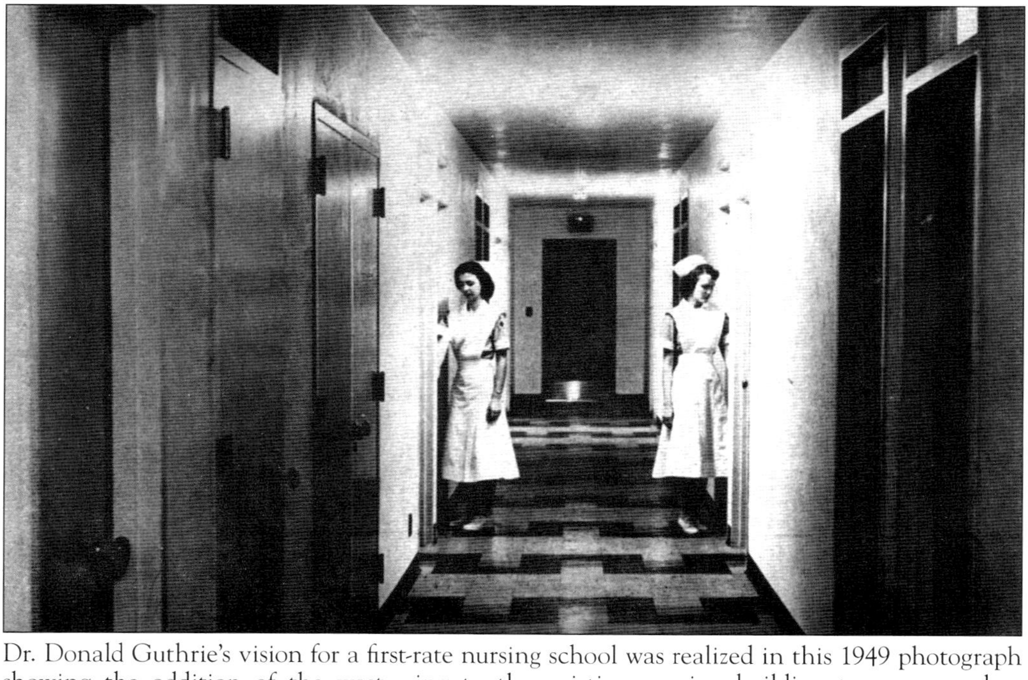

Dr. Donald Guthrie's vision for a first-rate nursing school was realized in this 1949 photograph showing the addition of the west wing to the existing nursing building to accommodate growing class numbers.

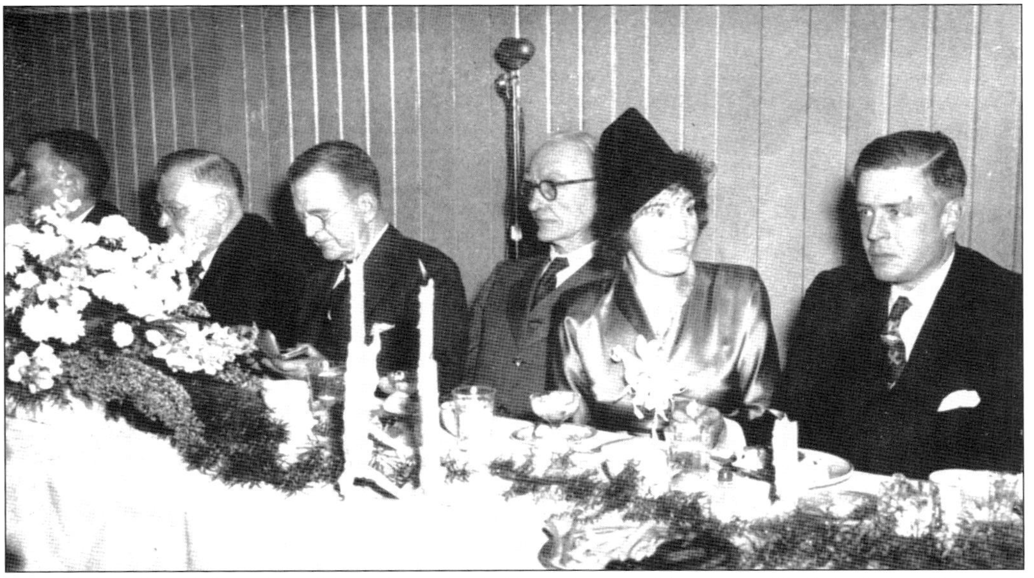

In 1950, Dr. Donald Guthrie (third from the left) was honored by the staff of Guthrie Clinic and Robert Packer Hospital for the 40 years he served as surgeon in chief. A clinical session was held in the afternoon, followed by an evening banquet attended by 250 friends and associates. At the meal, Dr. George W. Hawk said of Dr. Guthrie, "The many who know him cherish his attributes of character, personality, charm and his infinite capacity for sympathy and understanding, the greatest tribute we offer our chief is that he has inspired the deep love of his staff, present and past, and the many thousands of sufferers, to who, his presence, his word and his skill have given many hope and comfort and in many cases life itself."

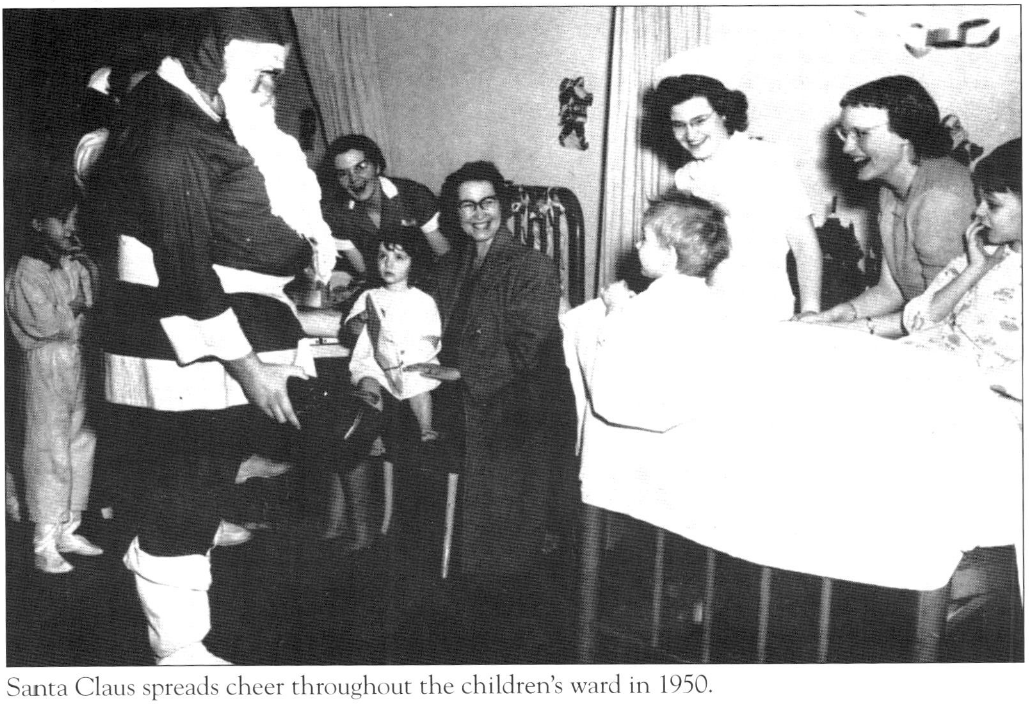

Santa Claus spreads cheer throughout the children's ward in 1950.

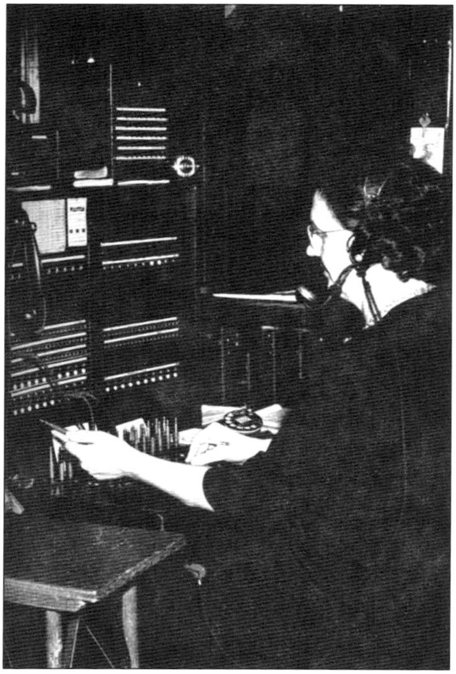

A great innovation, the new switchboard enabled operators to better handle calls in 1951.

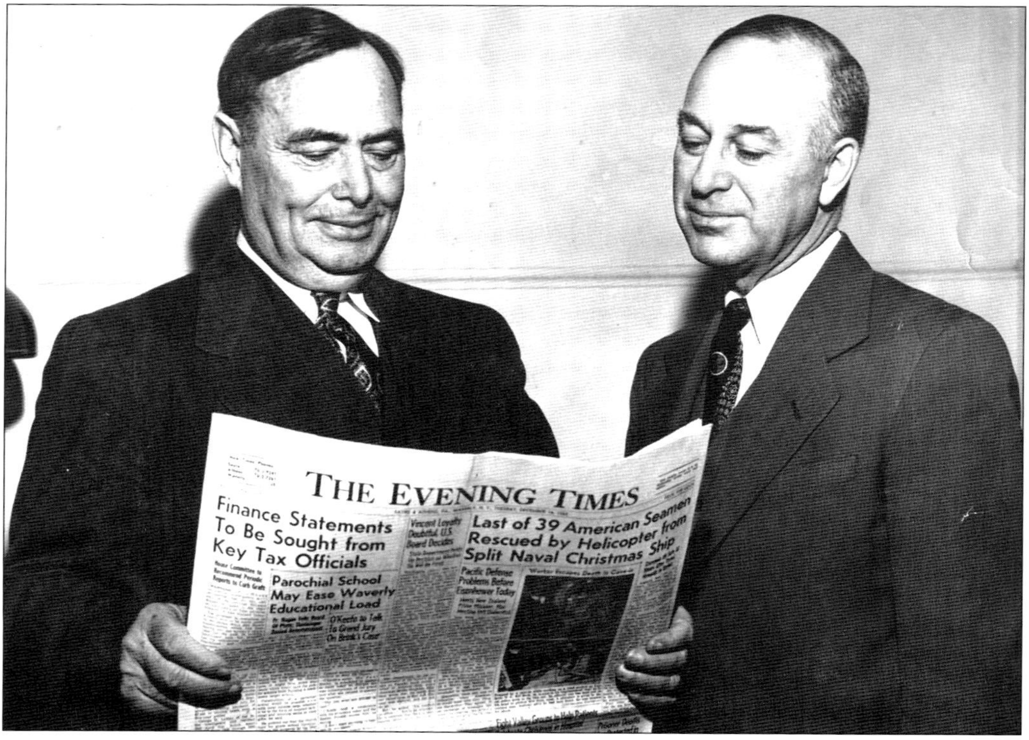
THE EVENING TIMES
Finance Statements To Be Sought from Key Tax Officials
Parochial School May Ease Waverly Educational Load
Last of 39 American Seamen Rescued by Helicopter from Split Naval Christmas Ship
Pacific Defense Problems Before Eisenhower Today

Speaker of the House Joe Martin (left) visits with Dr. Stanley D. Conklin in 1952. Martin was a Republican congressman from Massachusetts and was Speaker of the House twice, first from 1947 to 1949 and then from 1953 to 1955, when Dwight Eisenhower was president.

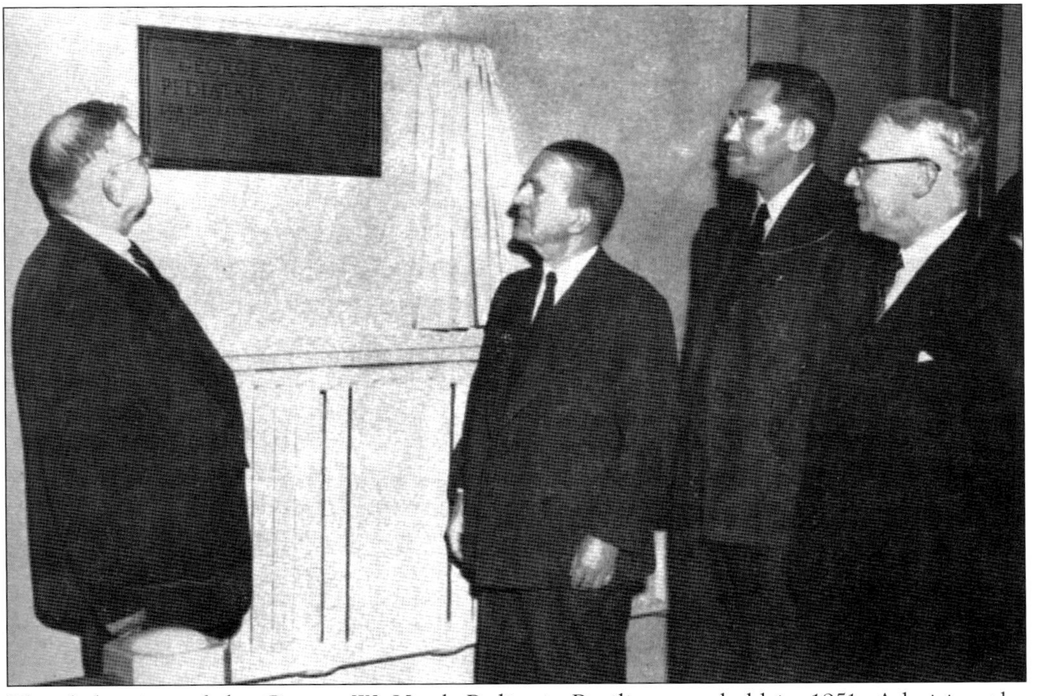

The dedication of the George W. Hawk Pediatric Pavilion was held in 1951. Admiring the plaque are, from left to right, Dr. George W. Hawk, Dr. Donald Guthrie, unidentified, and Dr. John M. Higgins.

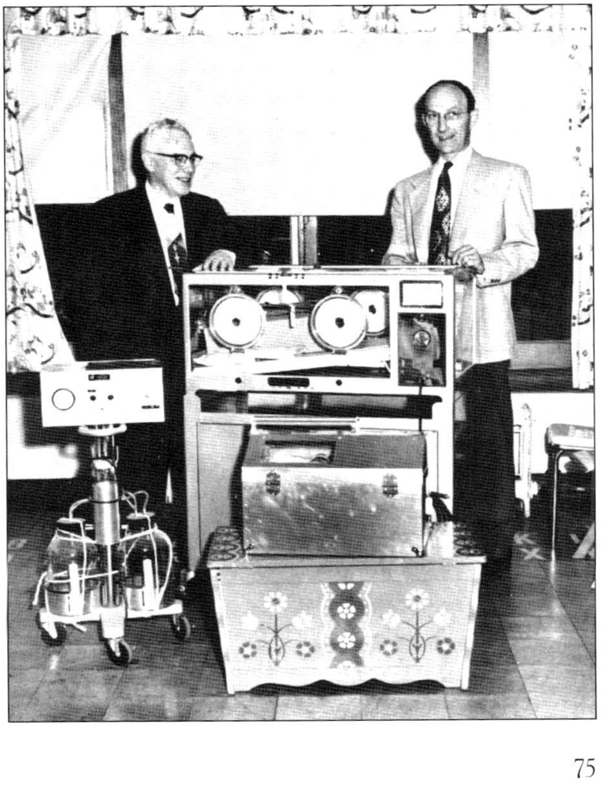

A testimonial dinner was held to honor Dr. John M. Higgins (left) on January 10, 1956. Devoted friends and patients gave gifts to the hospital on behalf of the physician. In the photograph, Dr. Higgins and Charles Haluska pose with some of the donations.

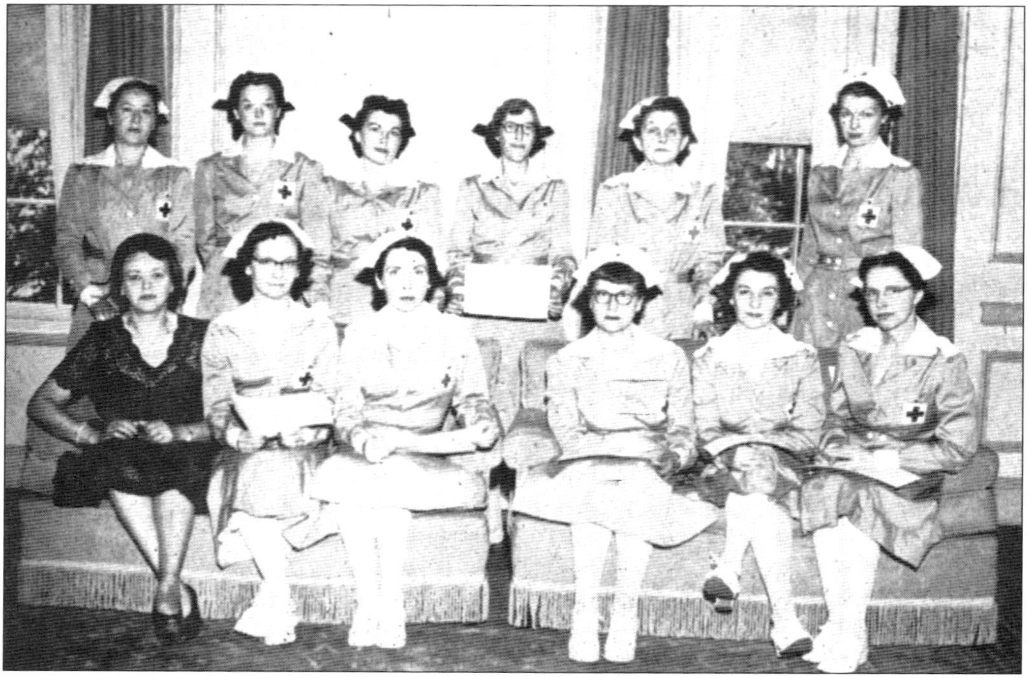

The Gray Ladies was the forerunner of today's volunteer department and was organized by Doris Rentschler (seated, third from the right), wife of Dr. Henry D. Rentschler. The ladies received training from the American Red Cross and did errands around the hospital.

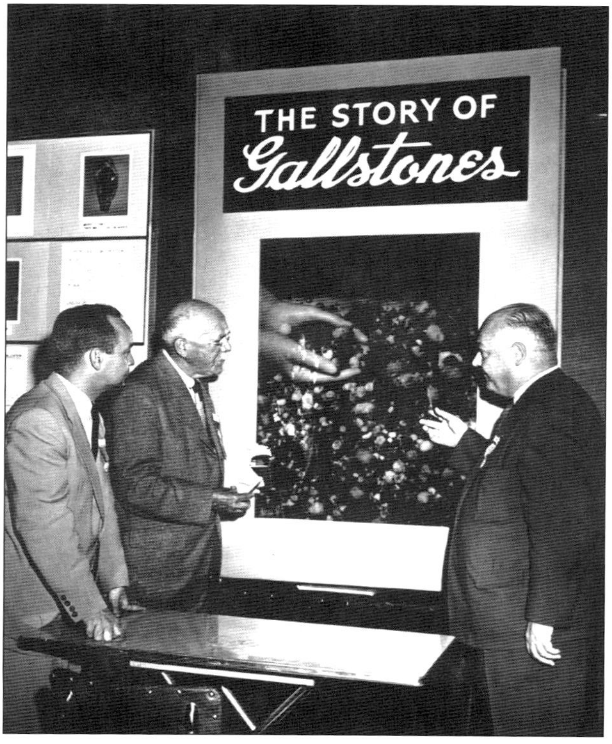

Dr. Donald Clough (far left) and Dr. Paul Shallenberger (right) pose next to Guthrie Clinic's exhibit at the American Medical Association's annual session in San Francisco, California, in 1954.

Paul Henry was a darkroom technician at Robert Packer Hospital trained under the rehabilitation program of the Pennsylvania Council of the Blind. He and his guide dog are shown at work in the hospital in 1957.

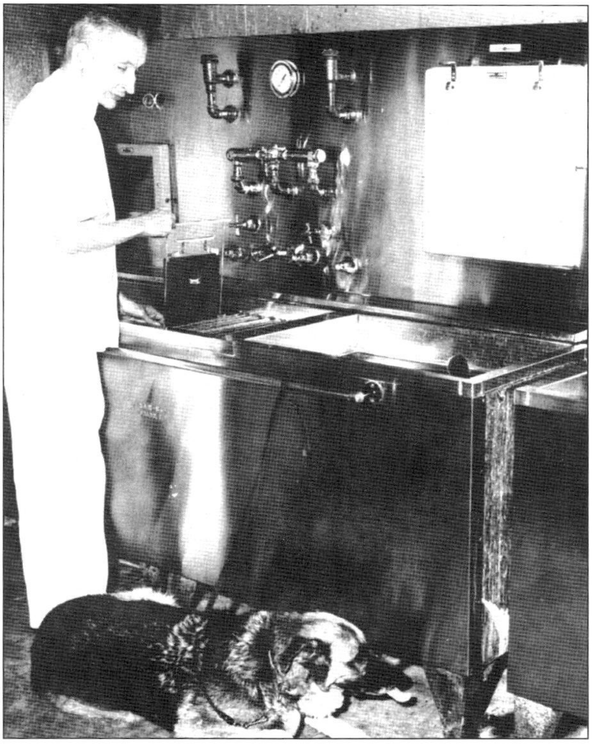

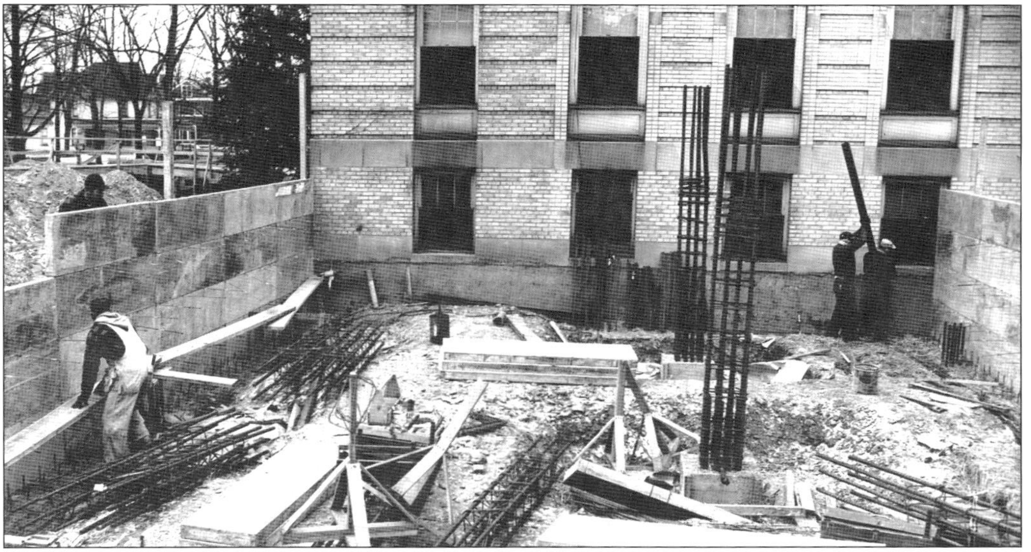

In 1956, a project adding new wings and a new lobby to the clinic building was completed. The new construction provided critically needed administrative areas, examining rooms for the doctors, increased laboratory facilities, a new staff auditorium, increased medical library space, a medical record area, and a beautiful lobby. Dr. Donald and Emily Baker Guthrie donated $20,000 for the lobby area and $800 toward the cost of lobby furniture. The clinic addition and rearrangement of the former clinic cost $508,563. The furnishings and office equipment were an additional $28,611.

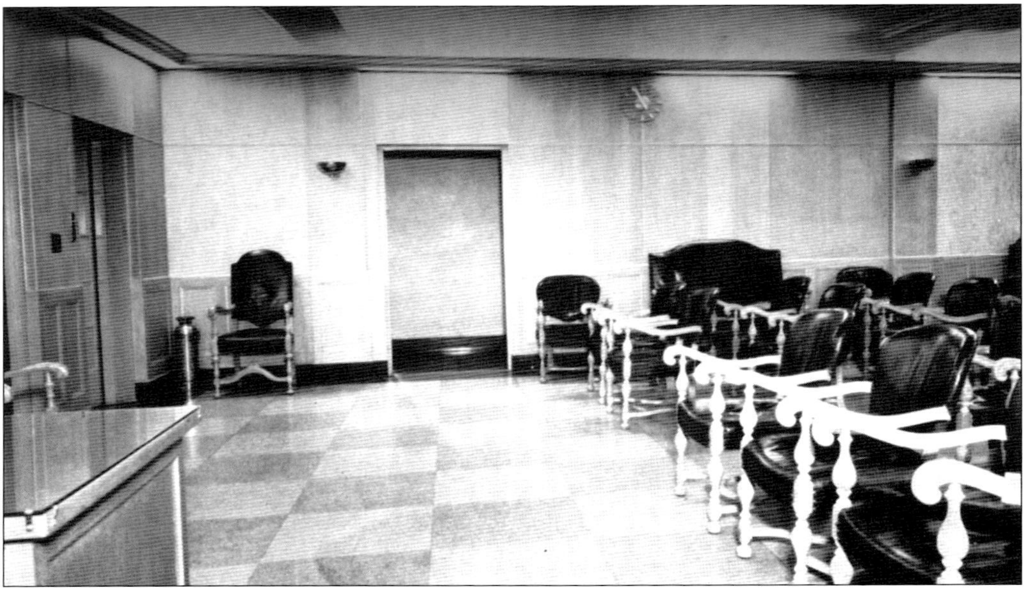

This photograph shows a remodeled waiting room in Guthrie Clinic.

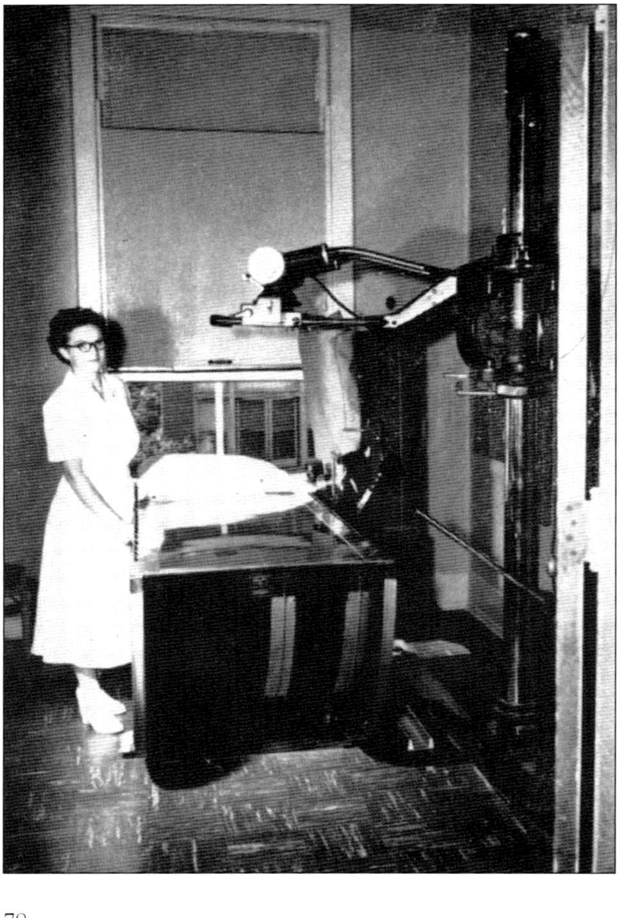

Continuing to offer the latest technology, a new Duoflex fluoroscopic X-ray machine was installed, shown here with Betty MacAfee, RT.

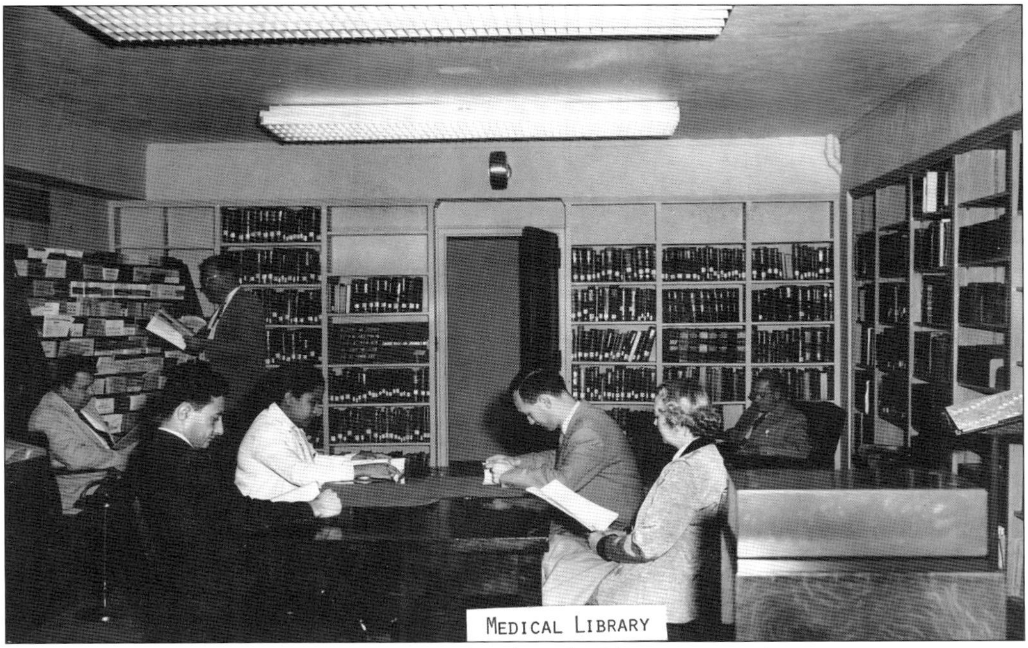

The medical library on the fourth floor of the clinic building continued to grow.

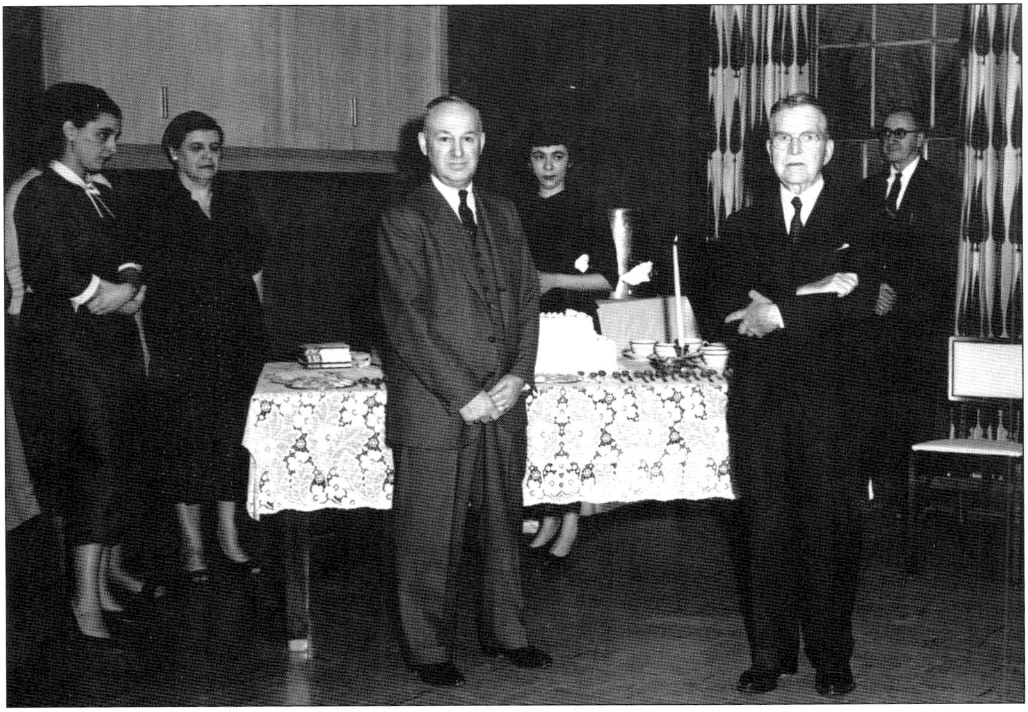

Friends, staff, and physicians honored Dr. Donald Guthrie on his 46th anniversary as a surgeon on January 10, 1956. Pictured are, from left to right, Margaret Lehr Wisniewski, librarian Barbara Cowley, Dr. Stanley D. Conklin, gift shop employee Charlotte Hafflet, Dr. Guthrie, and Dr. Charles H. DeWan.

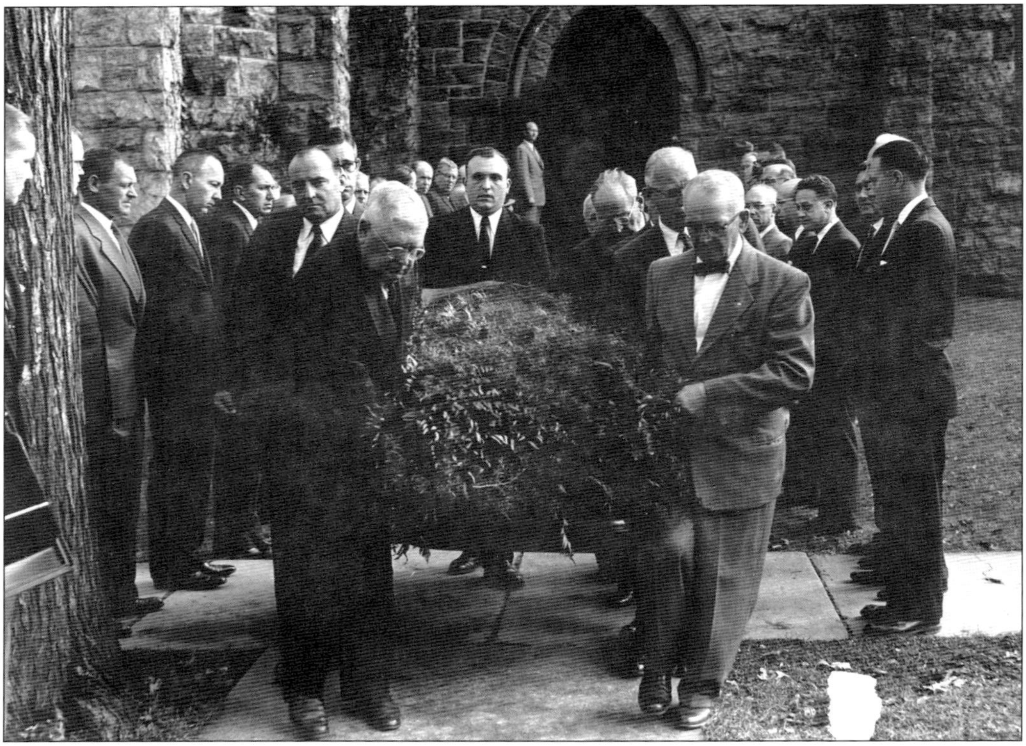

Dr. Donald Guthrie died at Robert Packer Hospital on October 30, 1958. His funeral was held in the Church of the Redeemer across the street from Guthrie Clinic. Pallbearers are, from left to right, Howard E. Bishop, Bird Sumner, Dr. Rodney L. Stedge, John Murray Jr., Dr. Malin Martin, Dr. Albert Murtland, Dr. Dominic Motsay, Dr. Gerard Gagon, and Dr. William C. Beck. All other Guthrie physicians were in an honor guard.

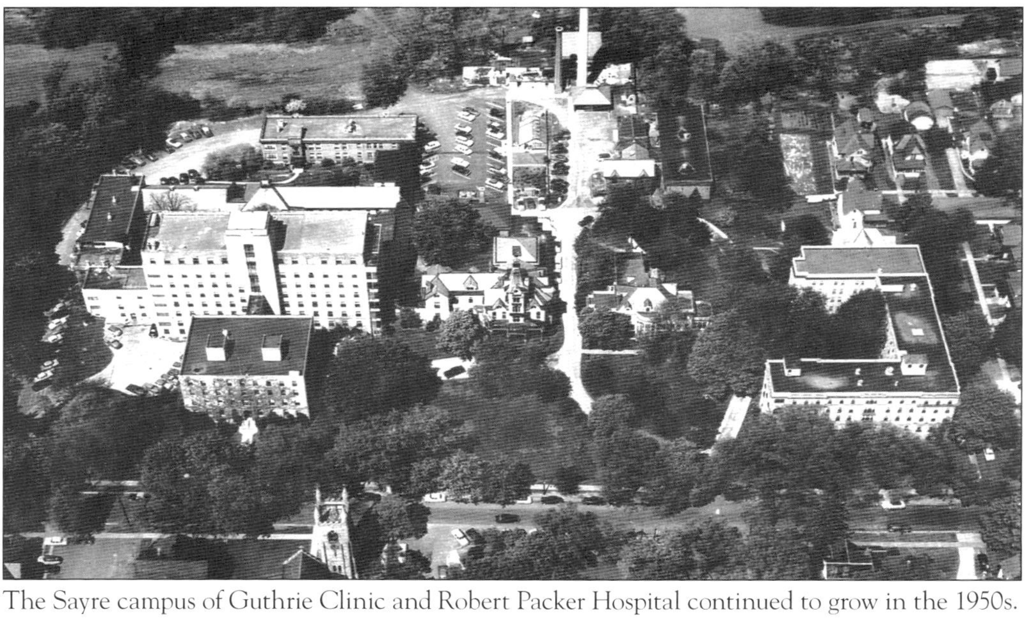

The Sayre campus of Guthrie Clinic and Robert Packer Hospital continued to grow in the 1950s.

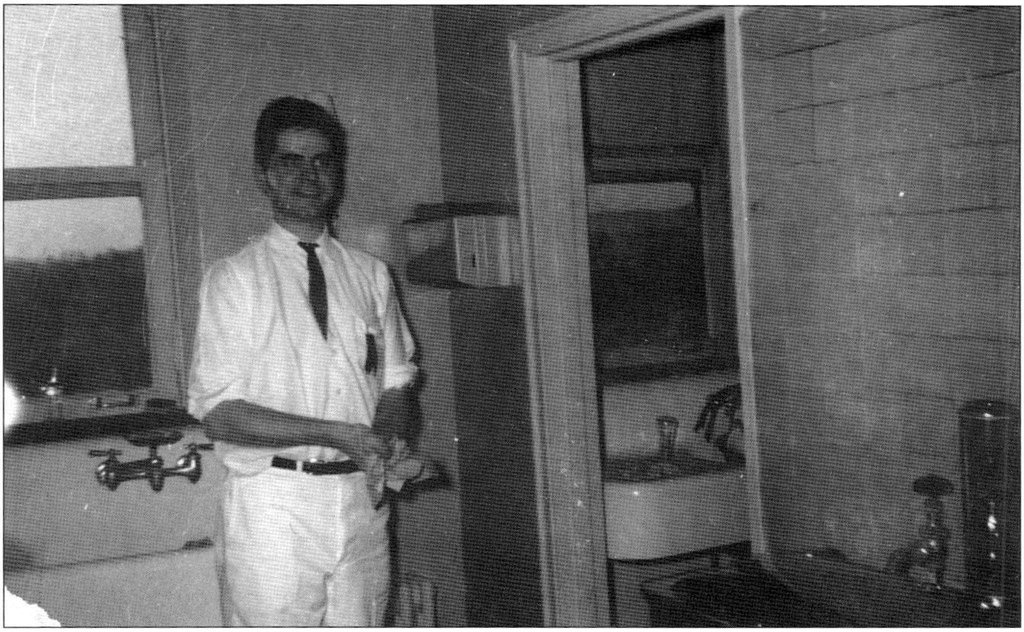

Dr. Charles H. Mayo II was an intern at Robert Packer Hospital from 1958 to 1959. He was the second generation of Mayo physicians to intern at Robert Packer Hospital. Interestingly, his son, Charles W. Mayo II, was born at the hospital on September 6, 1958.

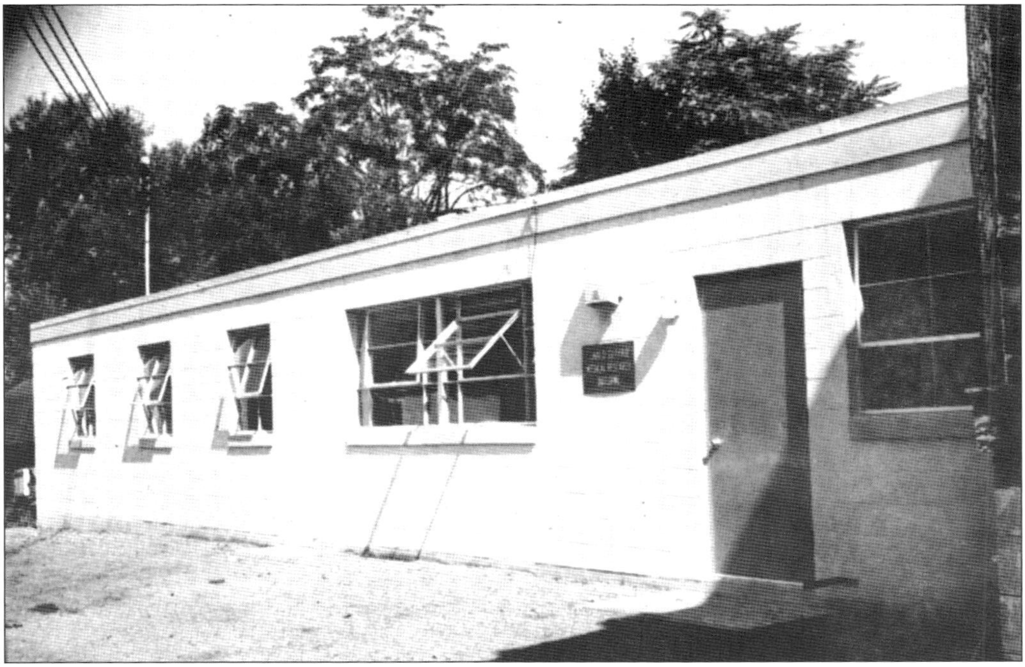

The Donald Guthrie Foundation for Medical Research, established by Dr. Guthrie in 1942 and chartered in 1944, was rebuilt in the 1950s. According to Dr. Guthrie, the hospital could not grow without a research arm to enrich and renew the ways it cared for patients. Emily Baker Guthrie's uncle Herbert Baker gave the first donation—$60,000.

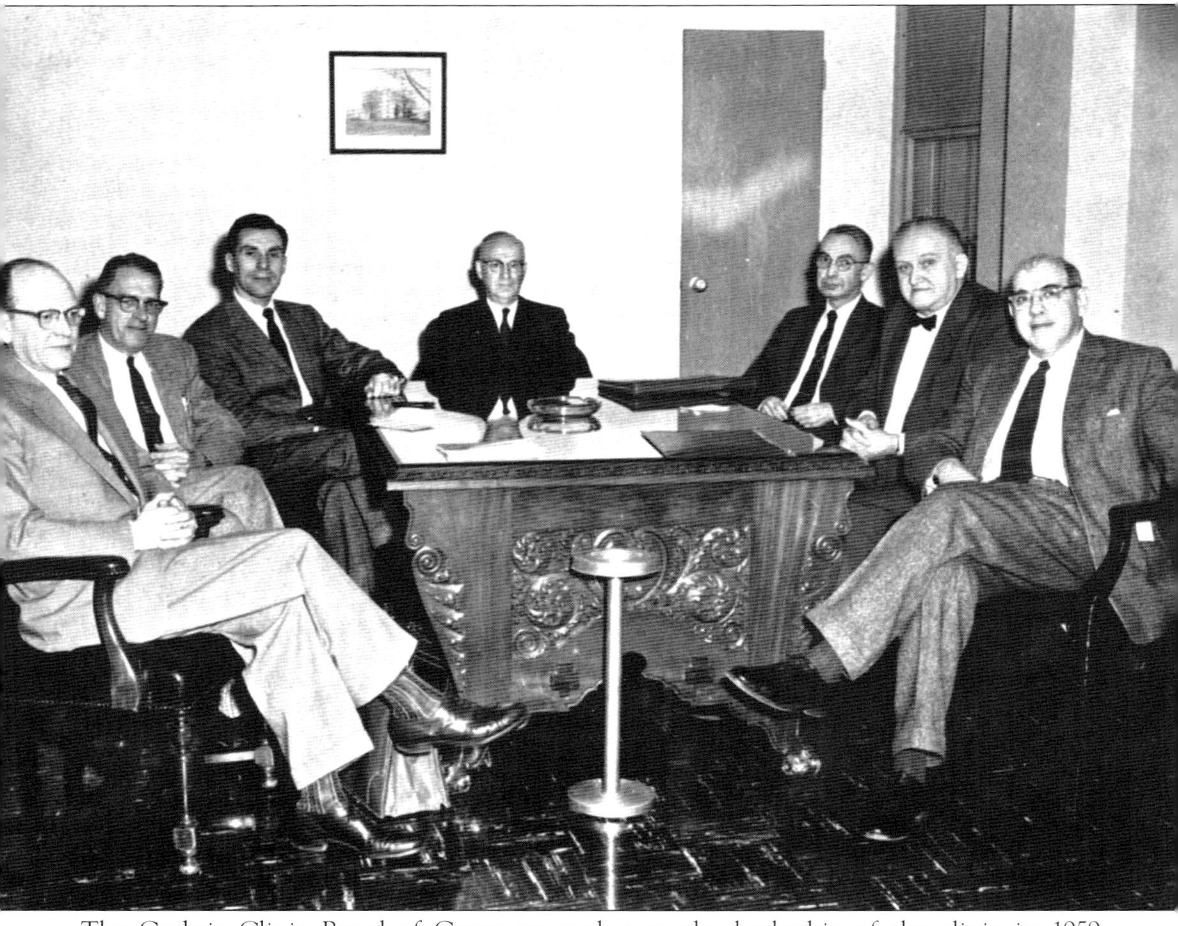

The Guthrie Clinic Board of Governors took over the leadership of the clinic in 1959 after the death of Dr. Donald Guthrie. Seated around Dr. Guthrie's desk are, from left to right, Dr. William F. Brehm, Dr. Joseph Cady, Ray K. Bolinger, Dr. Stanley D. Conklin, Dr. Henry D. Rentschler, Dr. William Baurys, and Dr. William C. Beck.

Seven

A New Generation

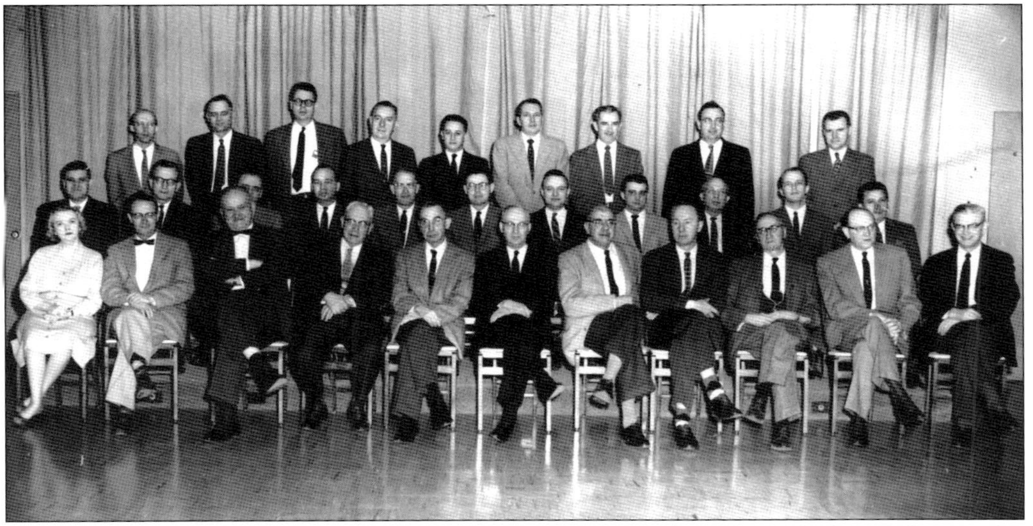

Pictured are senior staff of Guthrie Clinic and Robert Packer Hospital, from left to right, (first row) Dr. Virginia Whiteside, Dr. Jesse Littleton, Dr. William Baurys, Dr. John Higgins, Dr. Henry D. Rentschler, Dr. Stanley D. Conklin, Dr. William C. Beck, Dr. Edward Kulczycki, Dr. Charles DeWan, Dr. William F. Brehm, and Dr. John Niles; (second row) Dr. Arthur King, Dr. Joseph Flatt, Dr. Harold Collings, Dr. Donald Clough, Dr. Joseph Cady, Dr. Ralph Winston, Dr. Bruce Wimer, Dr. David Knapp, Dr. Malin Martin, Dr. James Erickson, and Dr. Warner Carlson; (third row) Dr. Albert Murtland, Dr. Ralph Scott, Dr. James Steele, Dr. Dominic Motsay, Dr. Wayne Allen, Dr. James Flood, Dr. Henry Perry, Dr. F. J. McDermott, and unidentified.

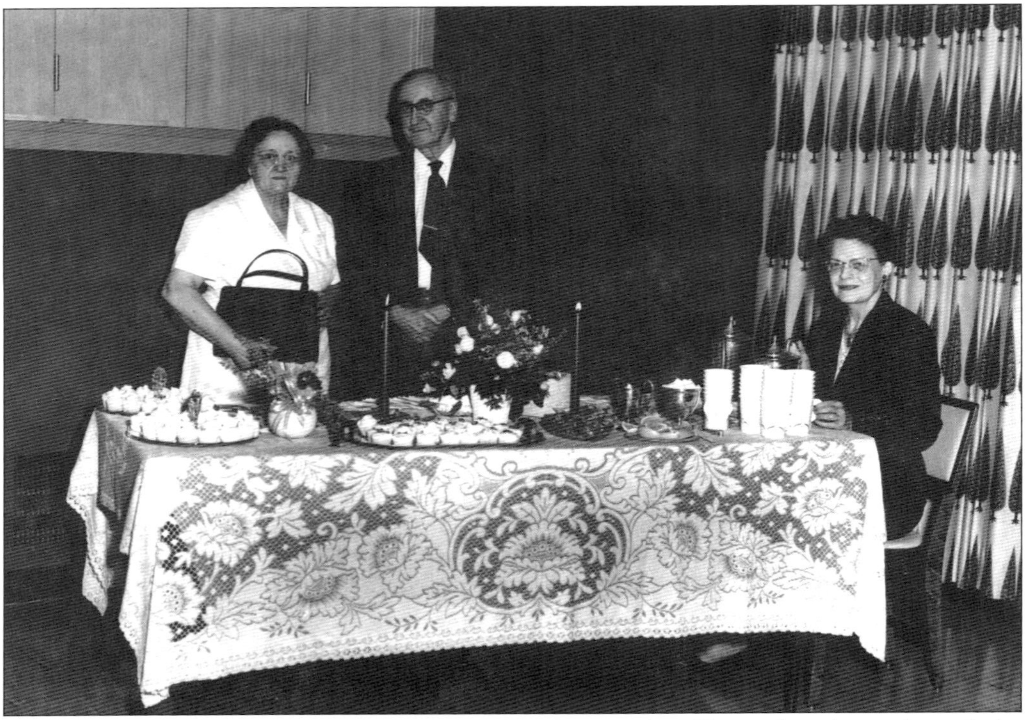

Isabell Setzer (left) was a longtime nurse at Robert Packer Hospital and member of the Robert Packer Hospital School of Nursing class of 1920. Dr. Charles and Ruth DeWan joined her at her retirement celebration.

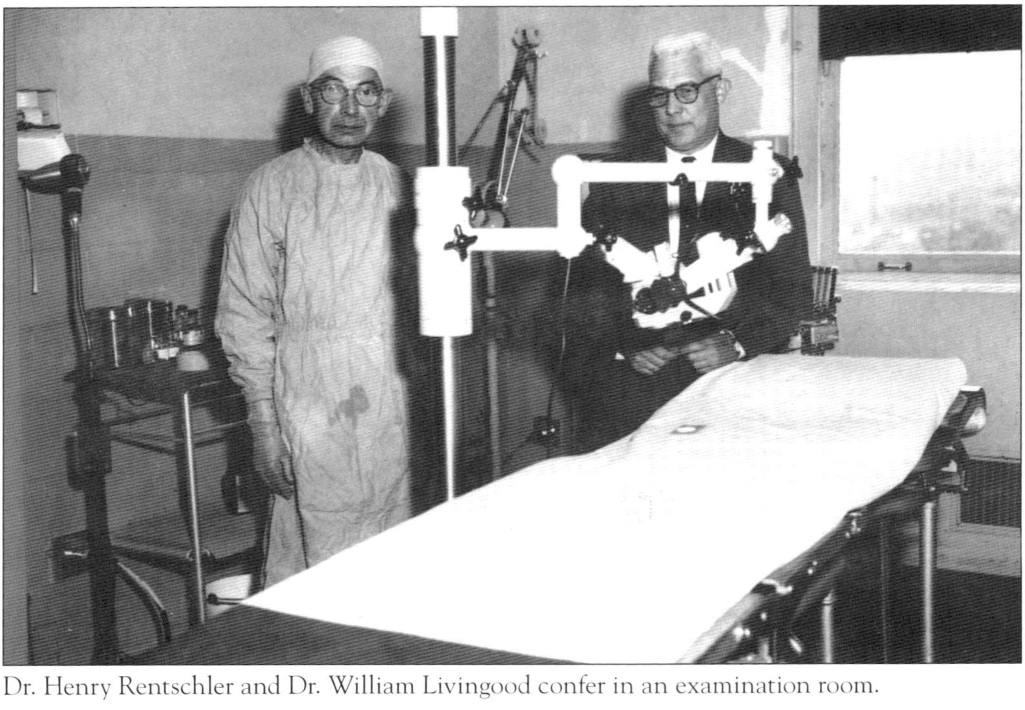

Dr. Henry Rentschler and Dr. William Livingood confer in an examination room.

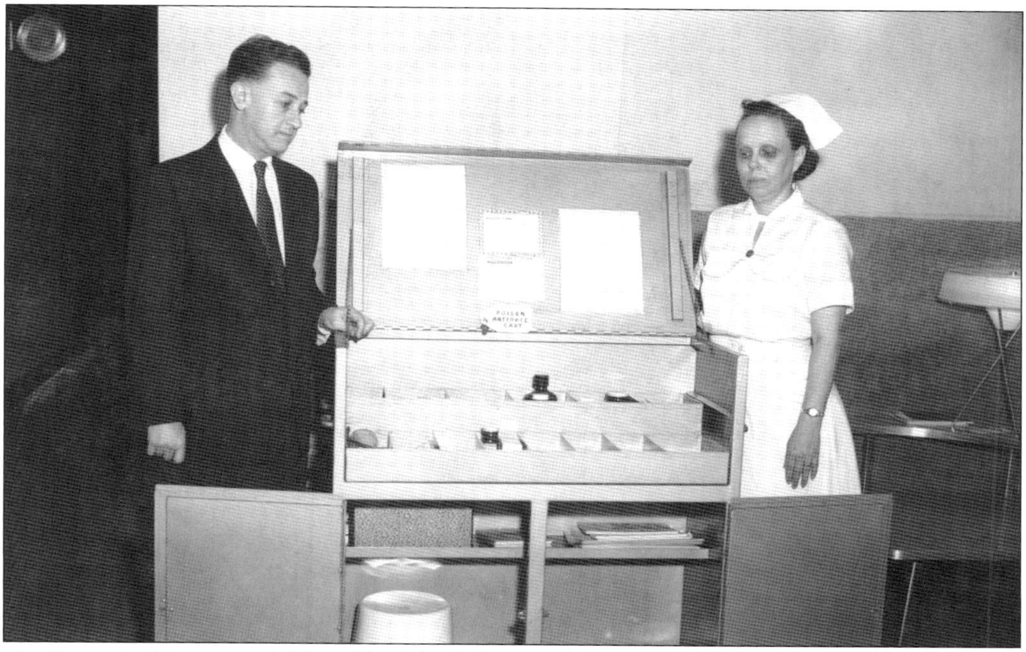

Dr. Dominic Motsay and Alice Skinkle, RN, reveal the contents of the poison antidote cart from the hospital's poison-control center, emergency outpatient department.

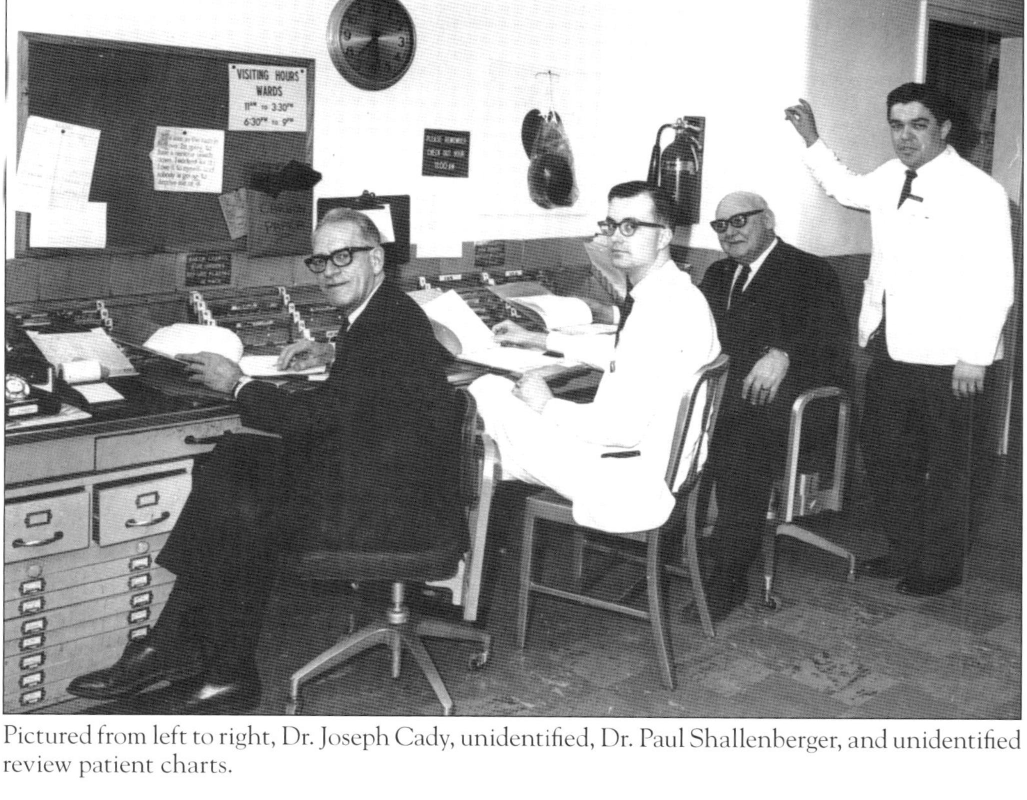

Pictured from left to right, Dr. Joseph Cady, unidentified, Dr. Paul Shallenberger, and unidentified review patient charts.

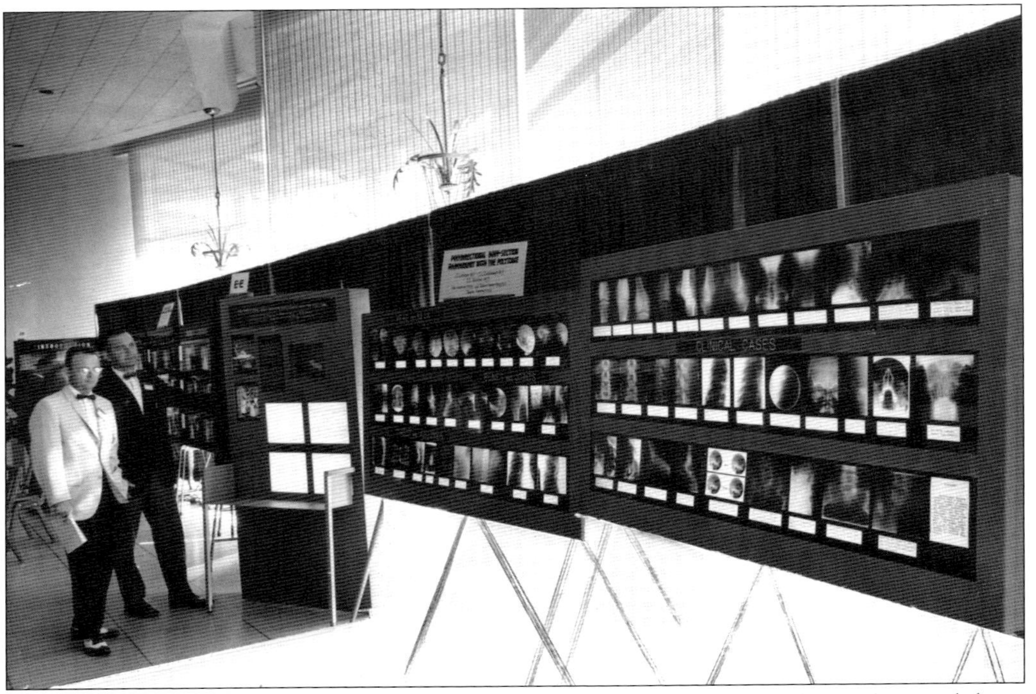

Dr. Jesse Littleton (left) and Dr. Fred S. Winter pose with a display highlighting the capabilities of the polydirectional body-section radiography with the polytome. Dr. Littleton used the first polytome in the United States at Guthrie Clinic in the 1960s.

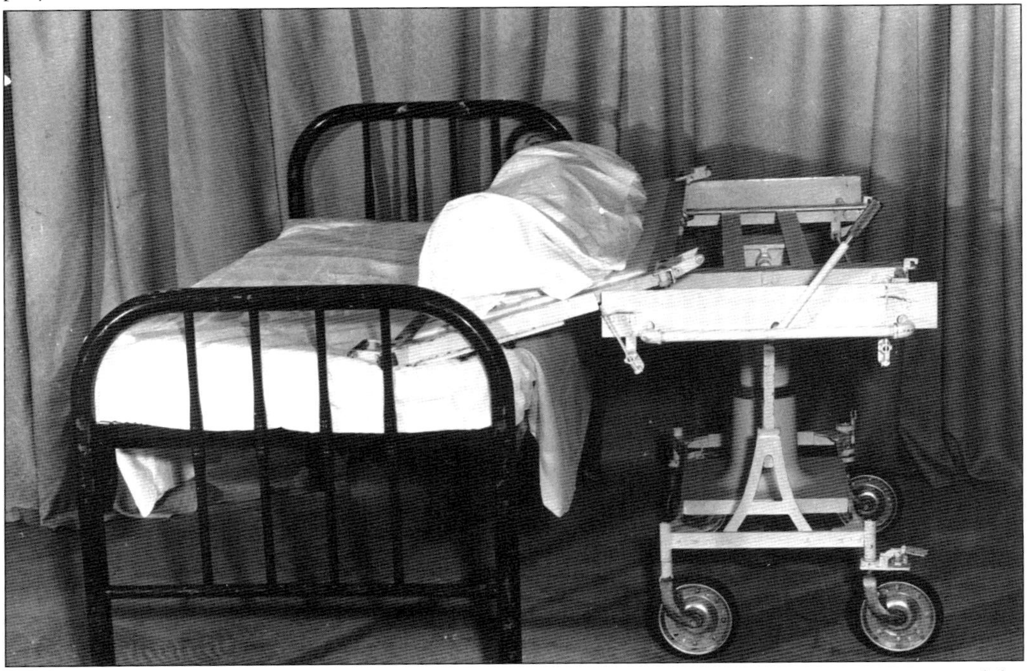

While at Guthrie Clinic, Dr. Jesse Littleton patented an innovative transport carriage used for the easy transfer of critically injured patients between their beds and diagnostic modalities.

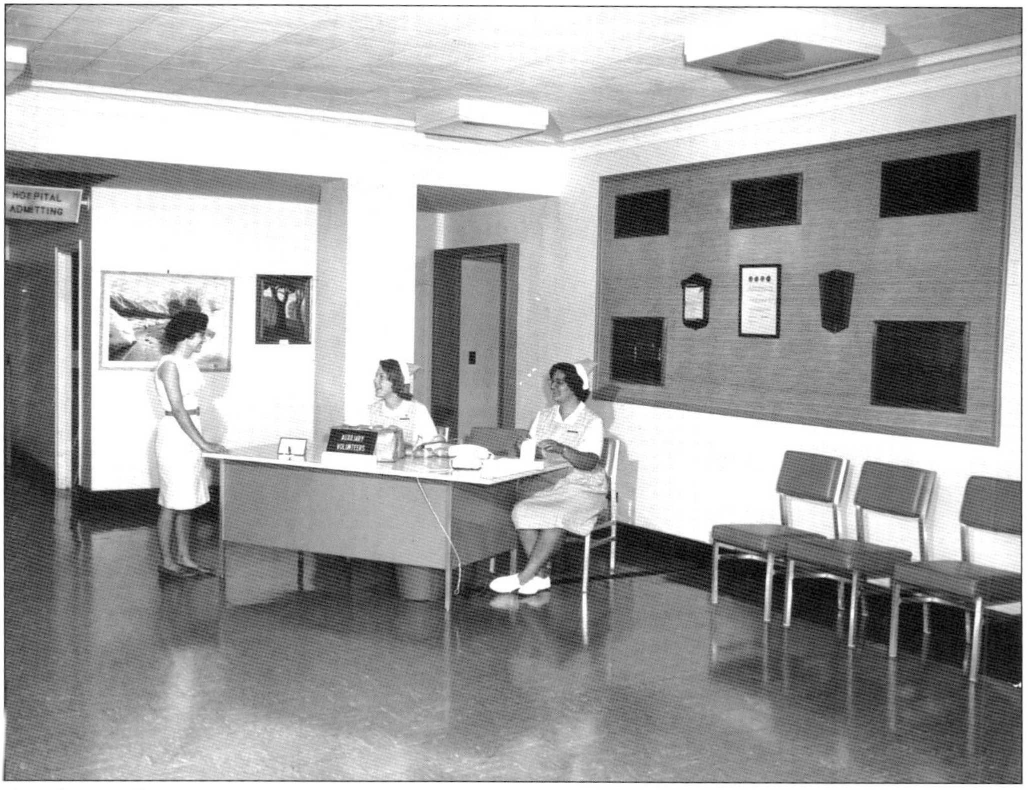

Auxiliary volunteers gather in the remodeled Guthrie Clinic lobby.

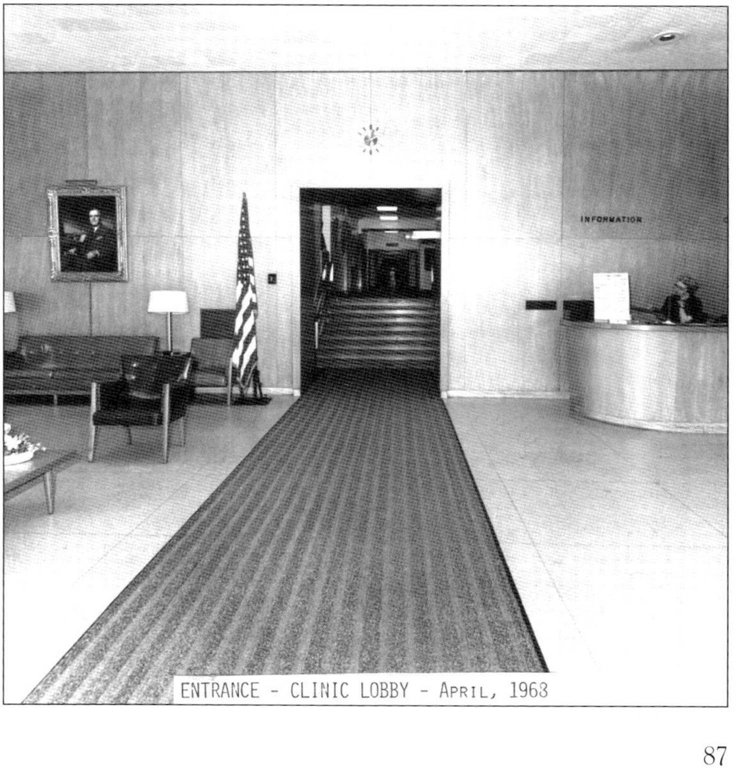

The entrance to the clinic and hospital is now the lobby of the Bird Sumner Building.

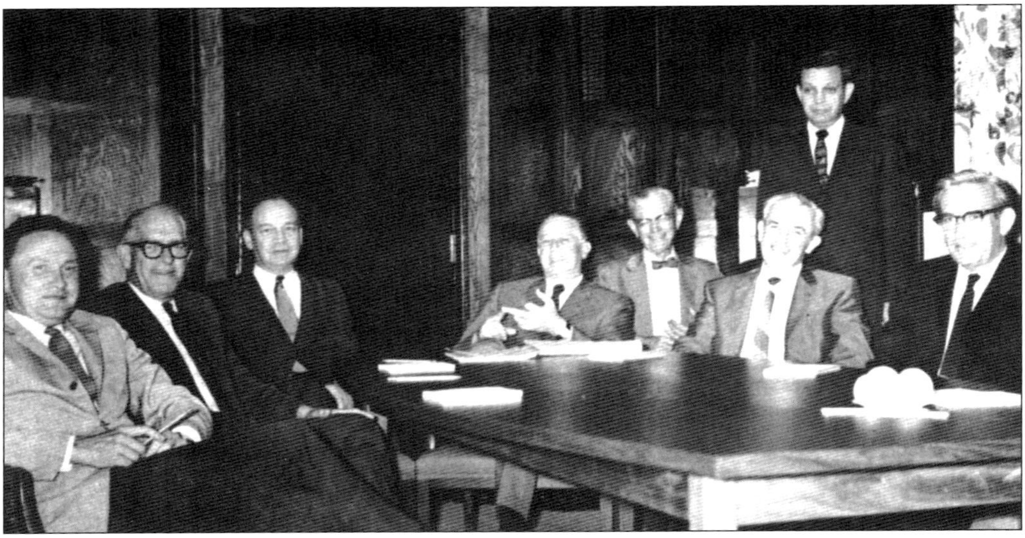

The Guthrie Clinic Board of Governors from 1969 included, from left to right, Dr. John Thomas, Dr. Joseph Cady, Dr. Donald Clough, Dr. Dominic Motsay, Dr. John Niles, Dr. James Flood, and Dr. Wayne Allen. Standing is clinic manager Harry Crandall.

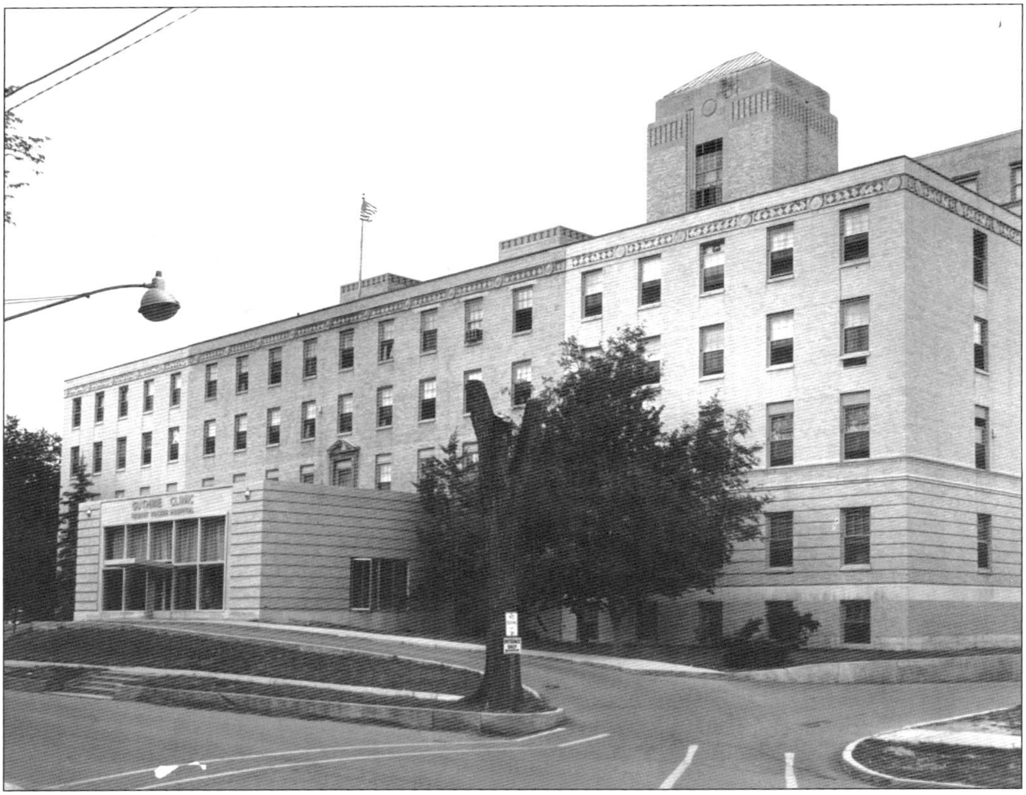

The Guthrie Clinic building in the 1960s is known as the Bird Sumner Administration Building today.

Eight

Becoming a Regional Medical Center

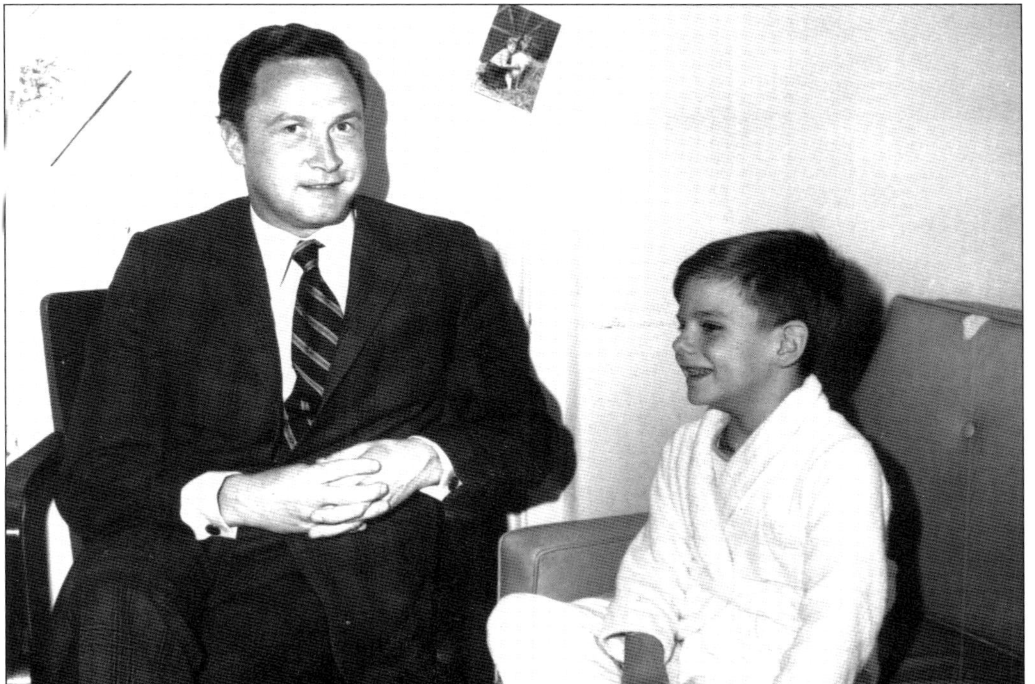

One of the more dramatic results of health care efforts at Guthrie Clinic occurred in May 1972, when a team of doctors led by surgeon Dr. John Thomas (left) saved a young boy's life by using an innovative blood "washout" procedure. The boy, Garth Shipman (right), fully recovered and visited staff at the medical center many times in the years afterward. The event was reported by national and international news media.

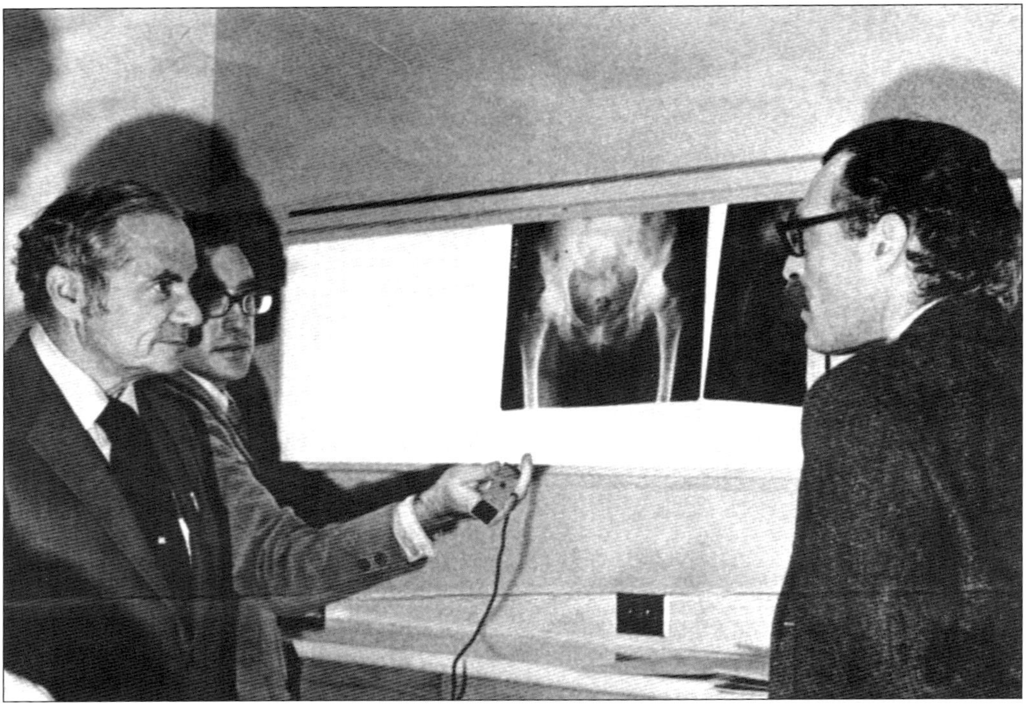

Dr. Bertram Bensam (left) explains the total hip operations being performed at Robert Packer Hospital to Pennsylvania governor Milton Shapp during a visit in 1972.

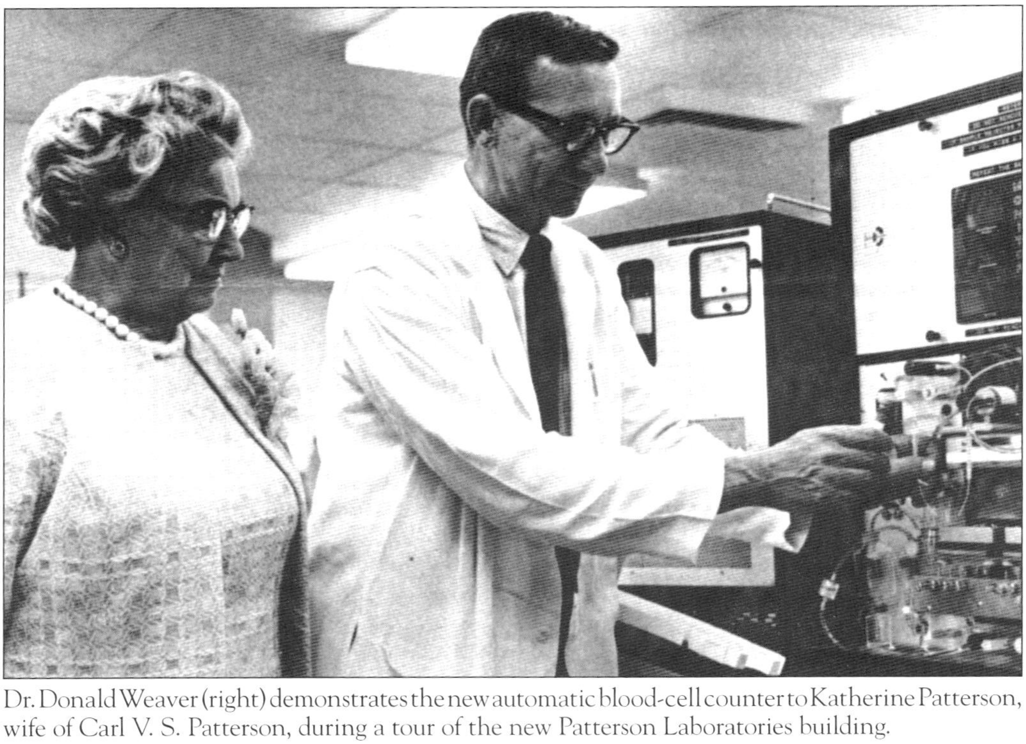

Dr. Donald Weaver (right) demonstrates the new automatic blood-cell counter to Katherine Patterson, wife of Carl V. S. Patterson, during a tour of the new Patterson Laboratories building.

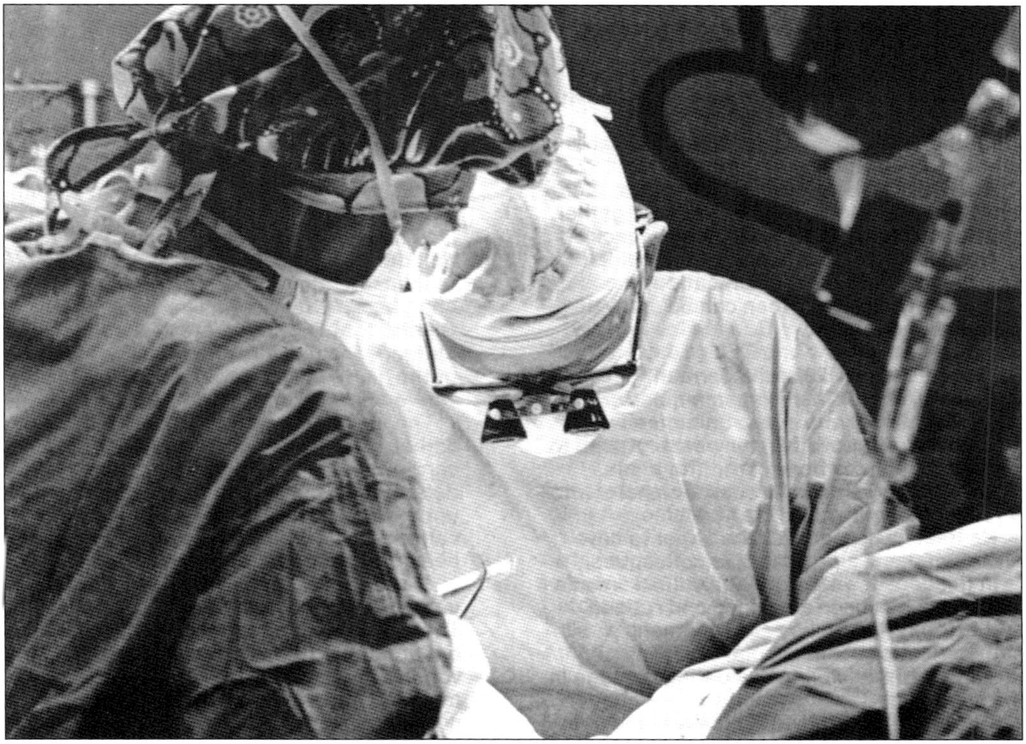

Dr. William Sewell, a pioneer in the surgical treatment of heart disease, was photographed here while performing an open-heart operation in the mid-1970s.

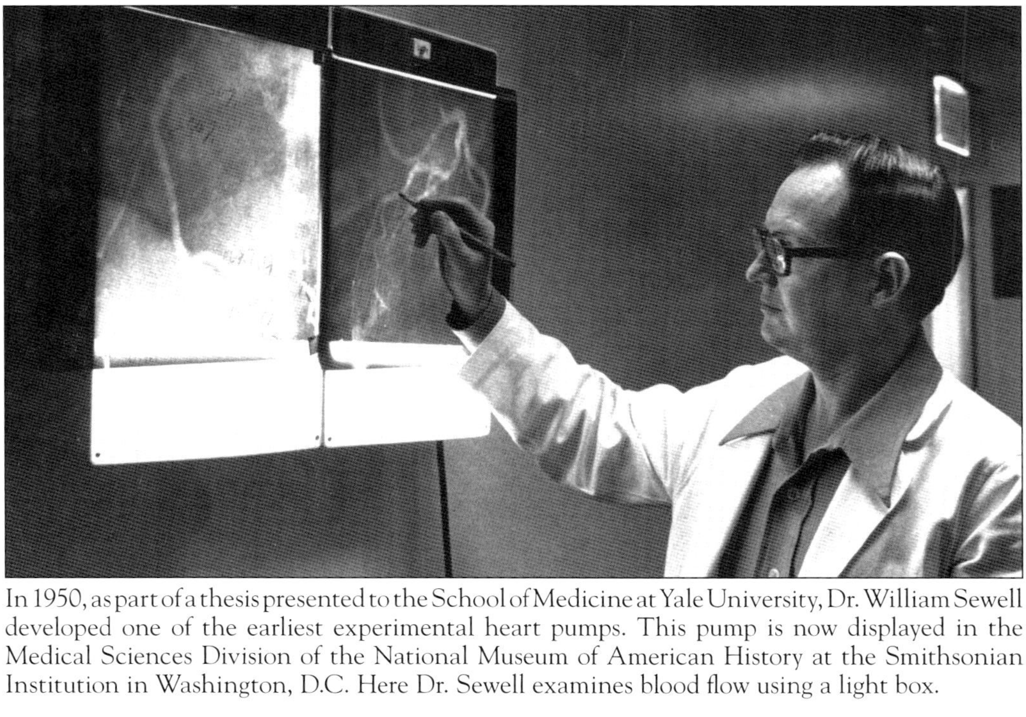

In 1950, as part of a thesis presented to the School of Medicine at Yale University, Dr. William Sewell developed one of the earliest experimental heart pumps. This pump is now displayed in the Medical Sciences Division of the National Museum of American History at the Smithsonian Institution in Washington, D.C. Here Dr. Sewell examines blood flow using a light box.

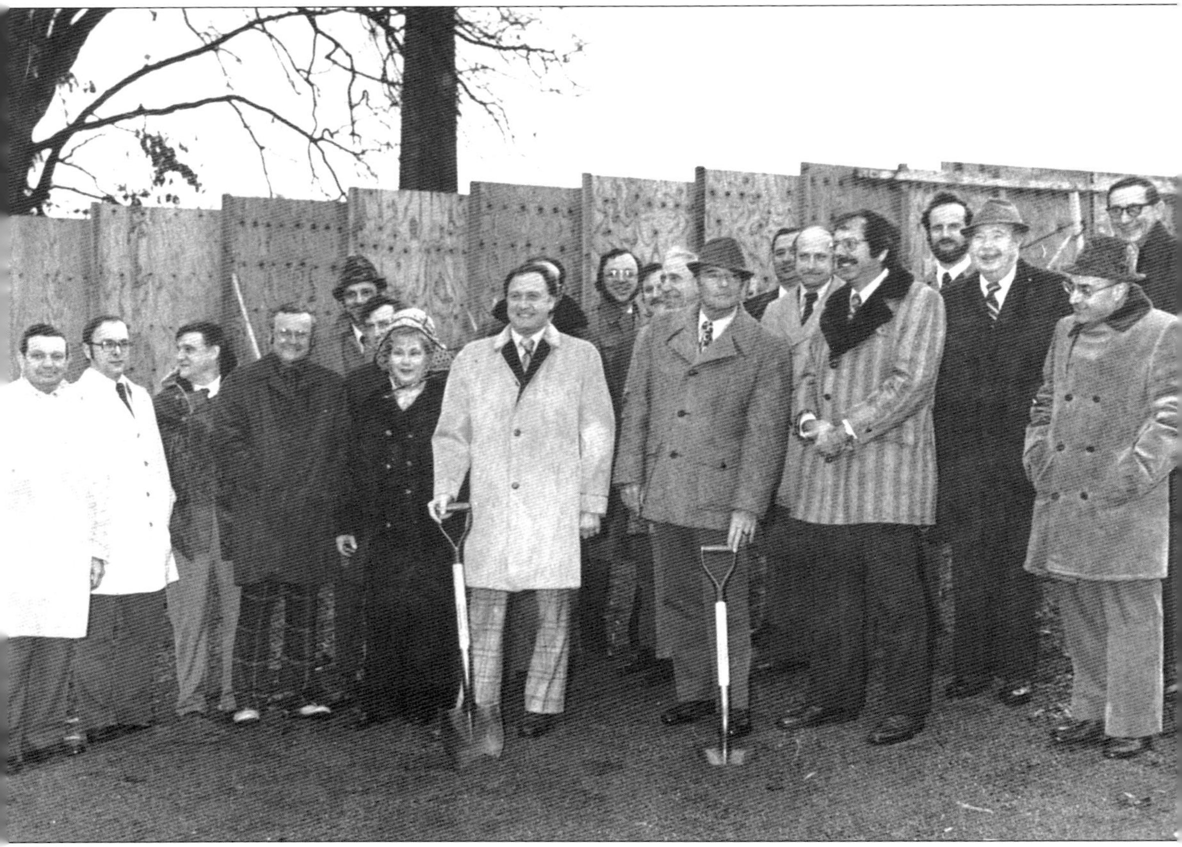

On May 19, 1975, a groundbreaking ceremony was held for new construction on the Sayre campus. In attendance are, from left to right, Harry Crandall, John Bailey, Dr. Arthur King, Dr. Bruce Boselli, Dr. Warren Nagle, David Gibbs, Betty Hasco, Dr. John Thomas, William VanSlyke, Walter Reick, Nicholas Chacona, Bird Sumner, William Cummings, Leo Wisniewski, Ralph Meyer, Dr. John Kelly, H. Slade Palmer, John Keiers, and Dr. Donald Weaver.

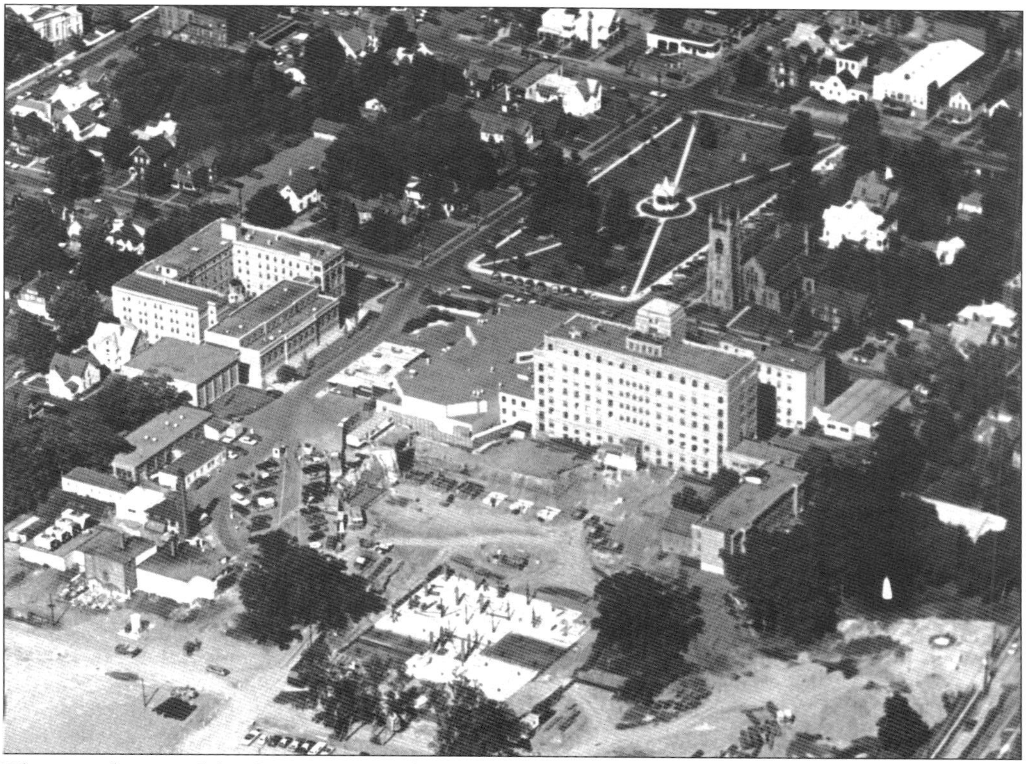

This aerial view of the Sayre campus shows the footers in place for the new clinic building.

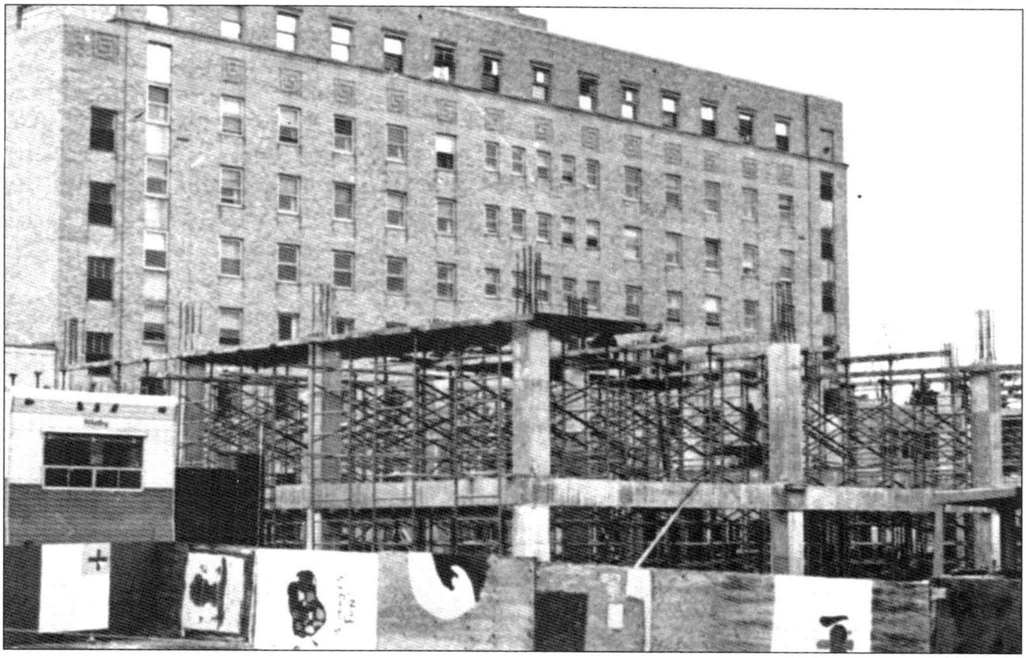

Another view of the Sayre campus shows the new construction of clinic and hospital buildings done in the 1970s.

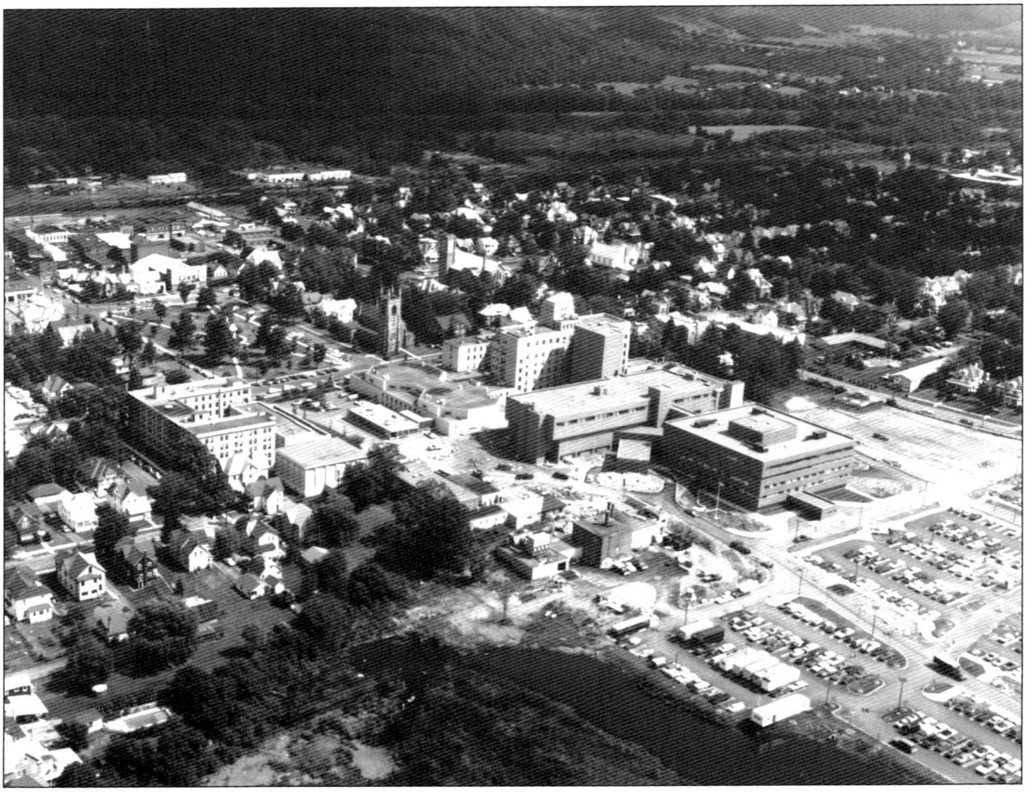

This photograph shows the recently constructed buildings for the clinic and hospital in 1977.

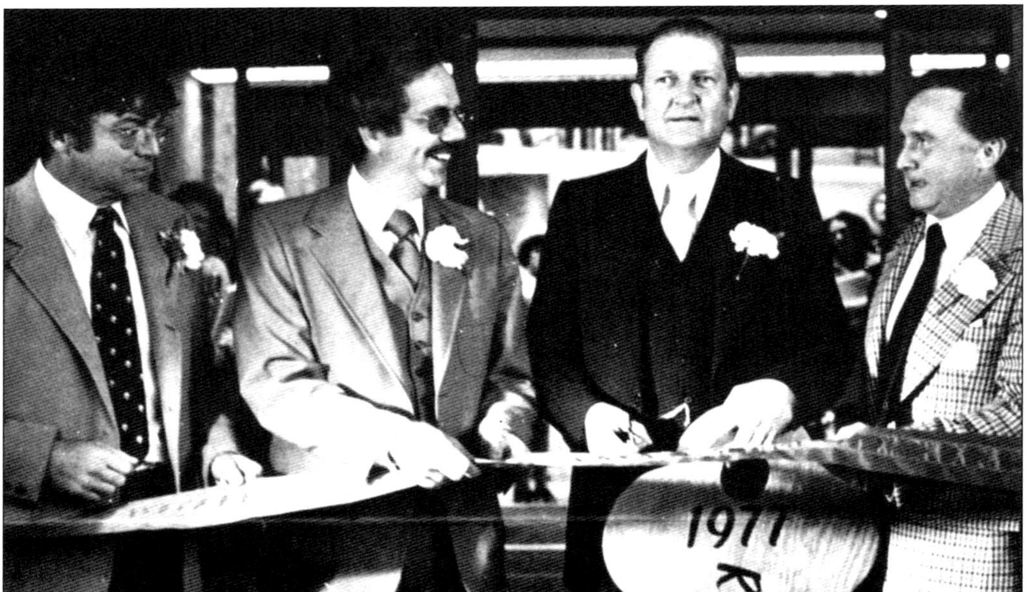

Officials from the hospital and clinic, from left to right, Dr. John Wanamaker, Ralph Meyer, Robert Landy, and Dr. John Thomas cut the ribbon to open the new facilities.

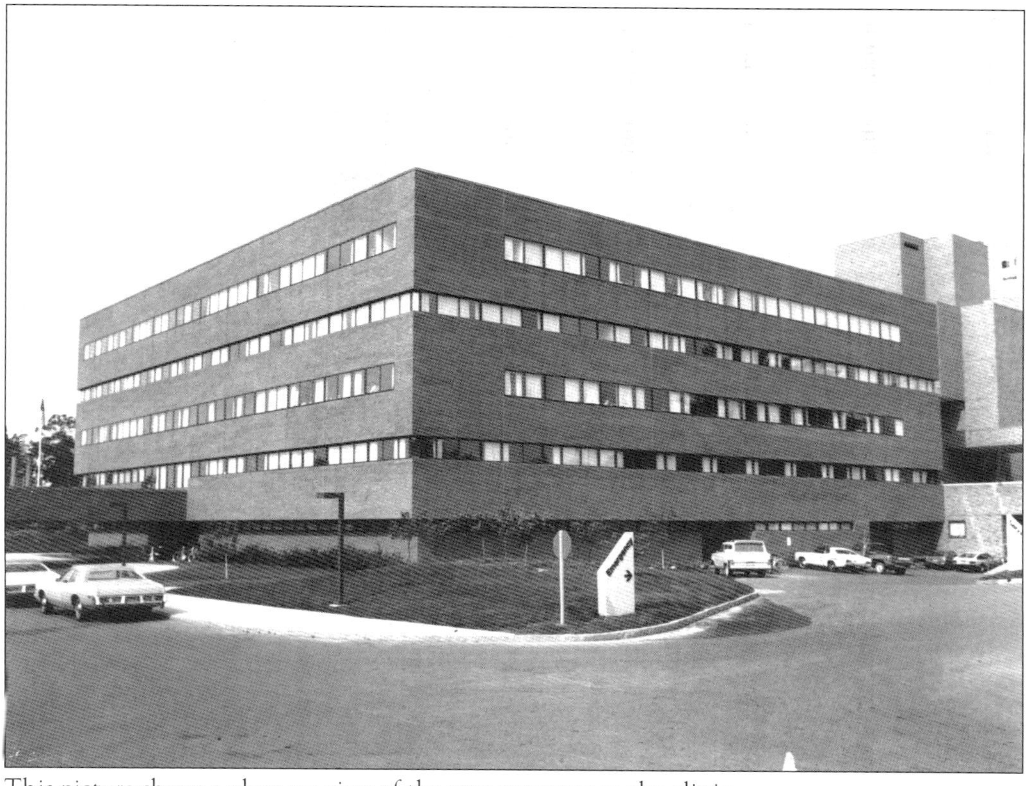

This picture shows a close-up view of the new entrance to the clinic.

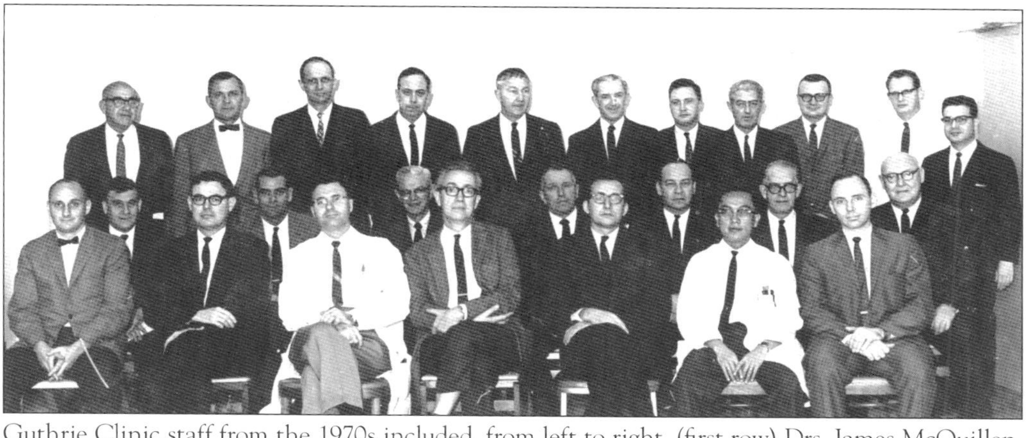

Guthrie Clinic staff from the 1970s included, from left to right, (first row) Drs. James McQuillen, Ralph Winston, Elliott Robinson, George Corner, Harold Liddle, Romulo Buano, and Bruce MacKay; (second row) Drs. Arthur King, Thomas Downey, John Niles, Wayne Allen, Donald Clough, Joseph Cady, and Paul Shallenberger; (third row) Drs. William C. Beck, Fred Winter, Warren Nagle, Robert Aronstam, Edward Kulczycki, James Flood, John Thomas, Jesse Carpenter, Bruce Boselli, and William Sewell. The physician on the far right is unidentified.

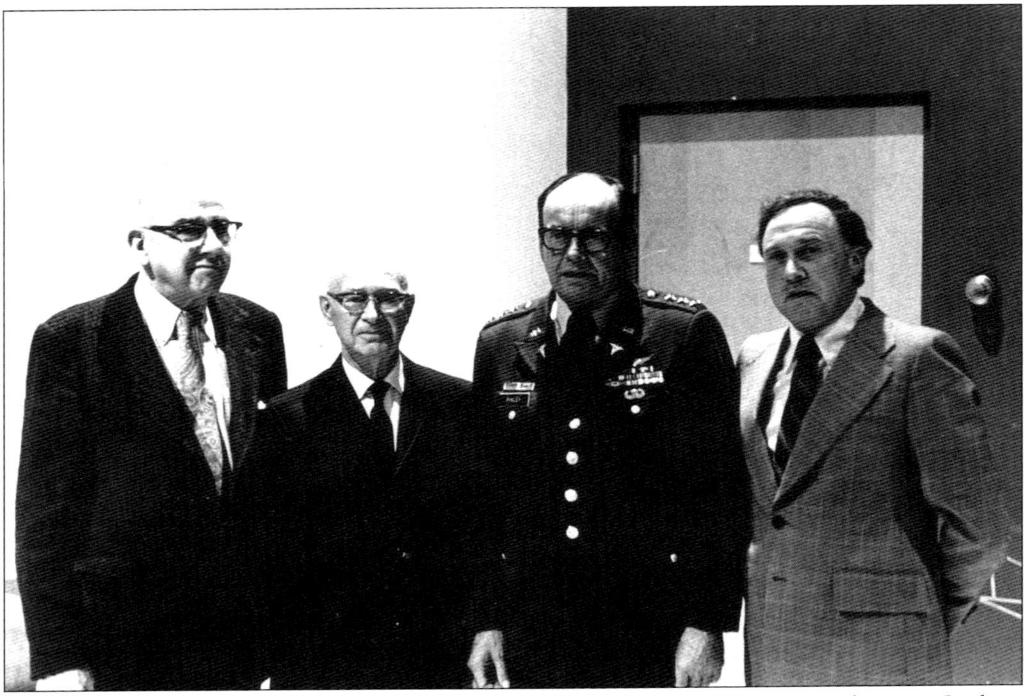

Former surgeon general of the U.S. Army, Charles Pixley was once a resident at Guthrie Clinic. Dr. Pixley (third from the left) is shown with, from left to right, Dr. William C. Beck, Dr. Stanley D. Conklin, and Dr. John Thomas during a visit to Sayre.

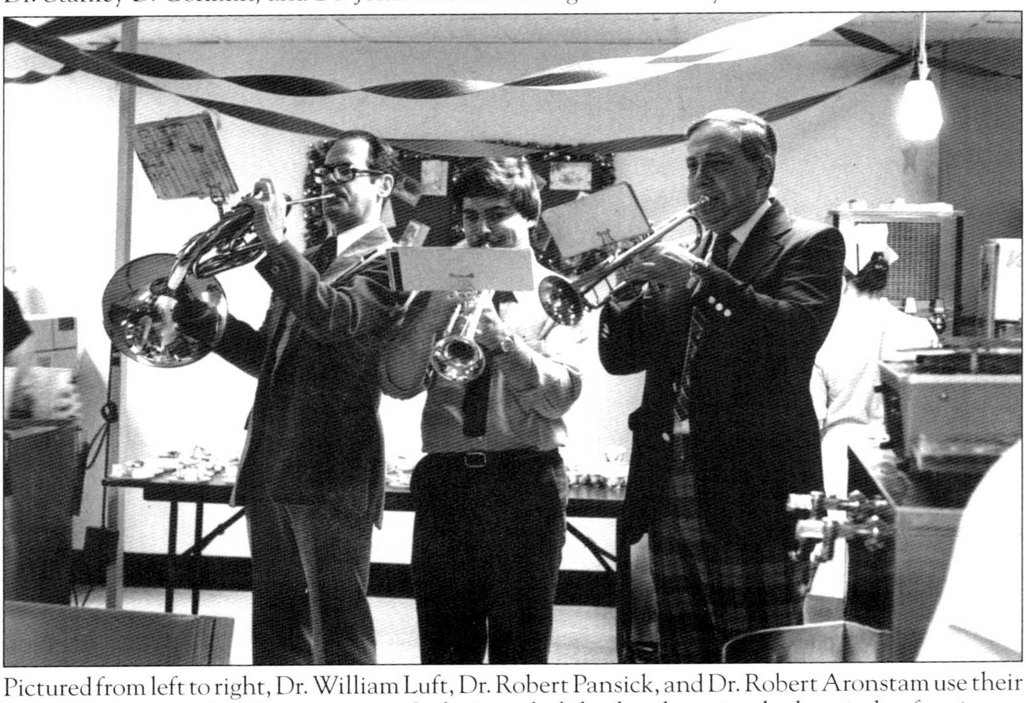

Pictured from left to right, Dr. William Luft, Dr. Robert Pansick, and Dr. Robert Aronstam use their musical talents to play Christmas carols during a holiday luncheon in the hospital cafeteria.

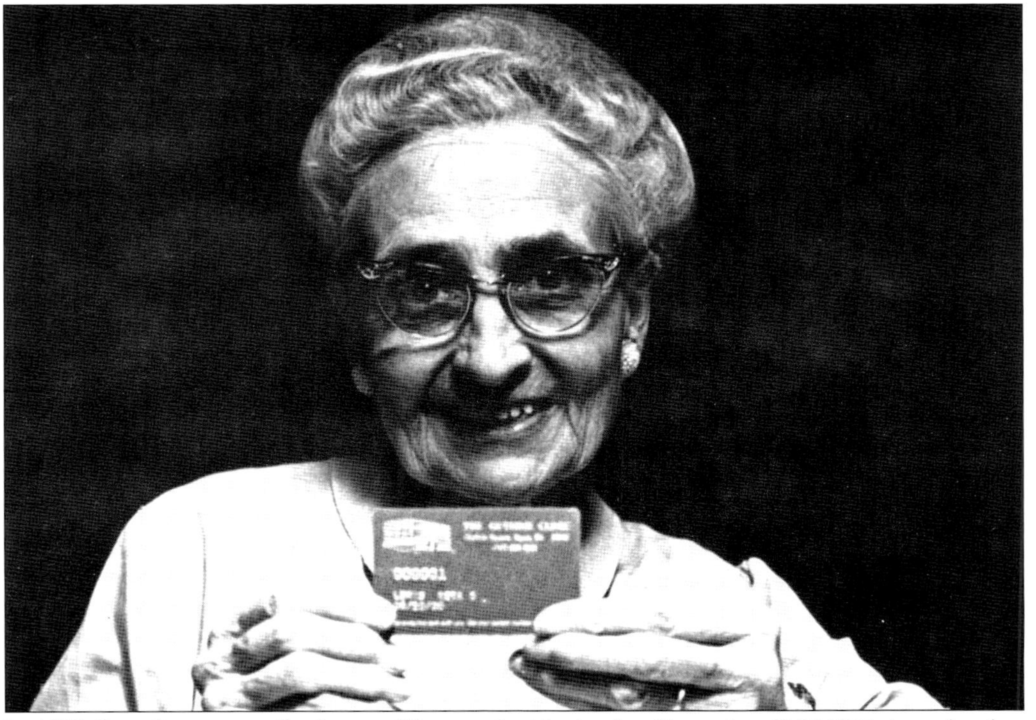

In 1978, Reta Lewis proudly shows off her card with the first B number, B 000001, issued to her on June 1, 1927, when she came to the hospital to have her third child. Six-digit B numbers were assigned to each patient as part of a medical record-keeping system after the original A numbers were retired from use.

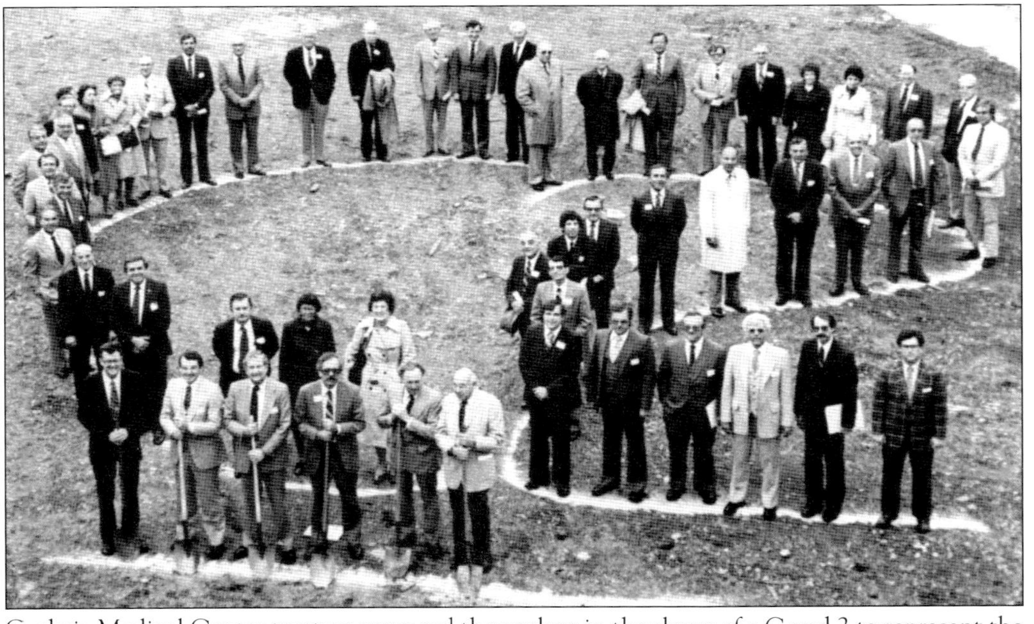

Guthrie Medical Center trustees arranged themselves in the shape of a C and 2 to represent the facility expansion undertaken in the early 1980s, known as the Century II building program.

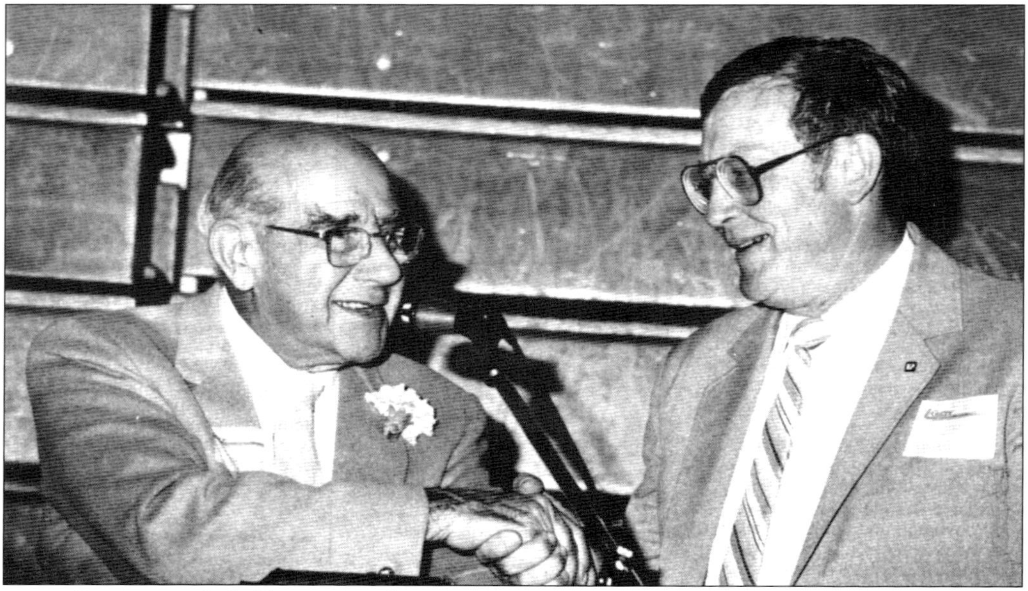

Dr. William C. Beck (left) receives a $100,000 check on behalf of the Donald Guthrie Foundation for Medical Research from IBM's George Houser.

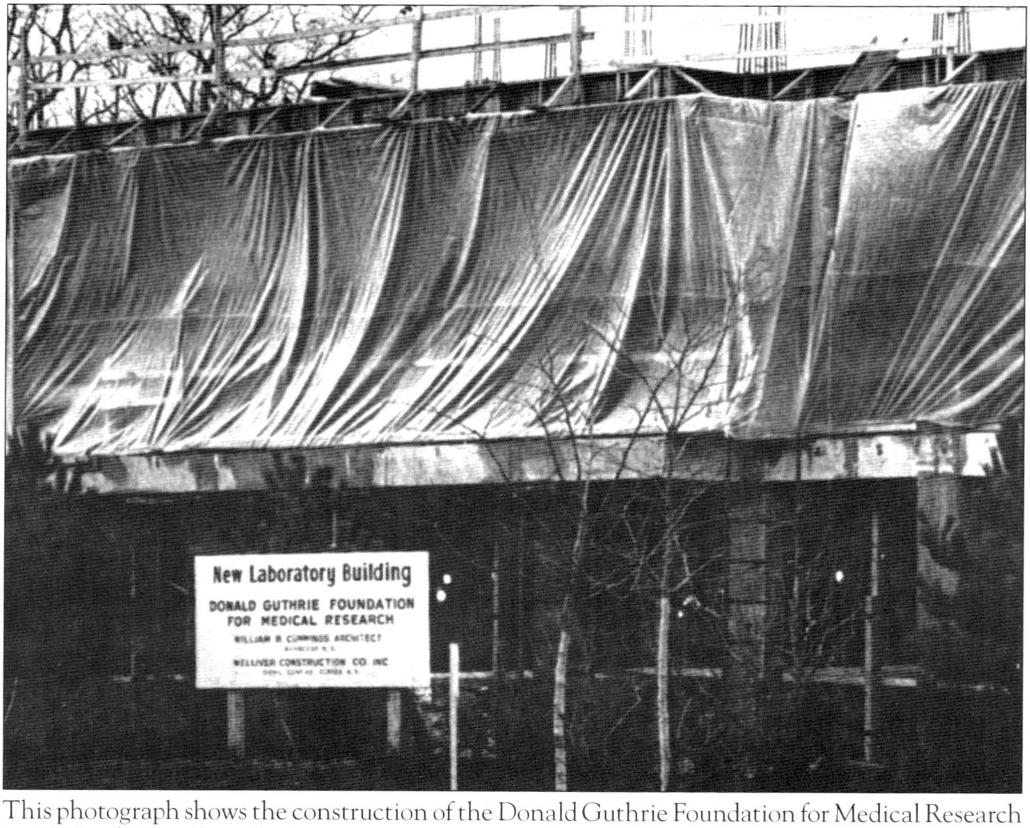

This photograph shows the construction of the Donald Guthrie Foundation for Medical Research in 1983, a $3.2-million facility.

Dr. Joseph A. Scopelliti, gastroenterologist, looks through the eyepiece of an endoscope in 1984. He had recently returned from a three-month stint in France training with Dr. Jean-Marc Brunetaud, an internationally renowned pioneer in the field of lasers.

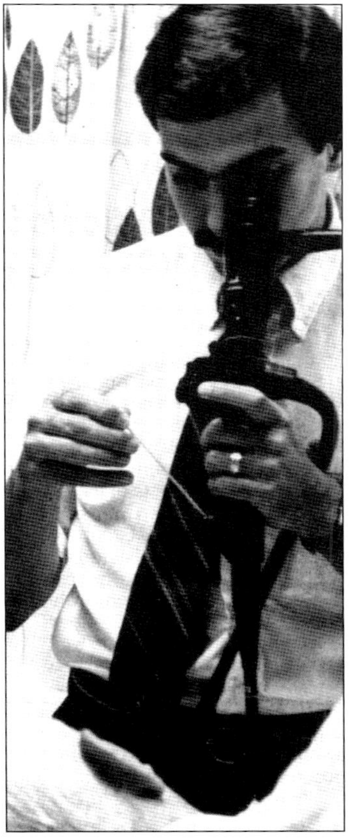

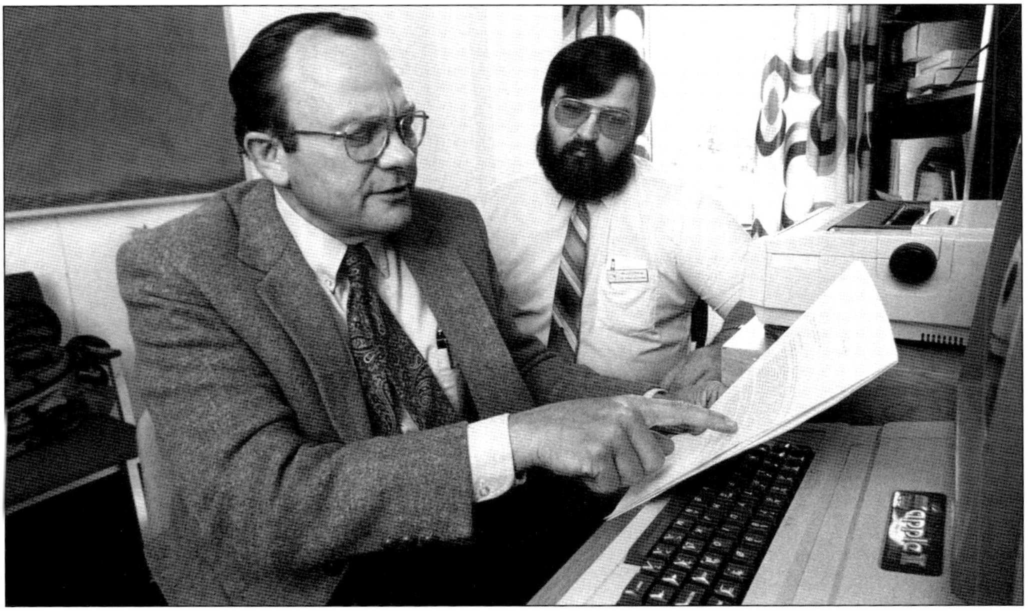

Dr. Ray Garman (left), pulmonary medicine, reviews a document with respiratory therapist Paul Chacona in 1985.

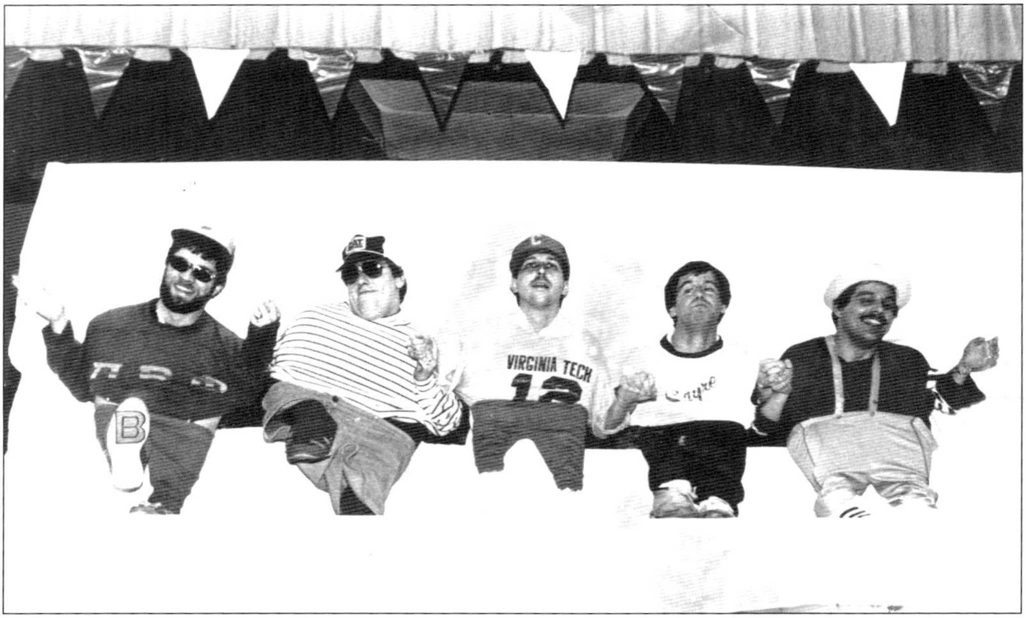

A circus was one of the events scheduled to celebrate the 100th anniversary of Robert Packer Hospital in 1985. The hit of the show was the hospital residents performing as the Little People. They are, from left to right, Bill Iobst, Jon Sorber, Doug Kirtley, Bob Yamulla, and Bill Namestnik.

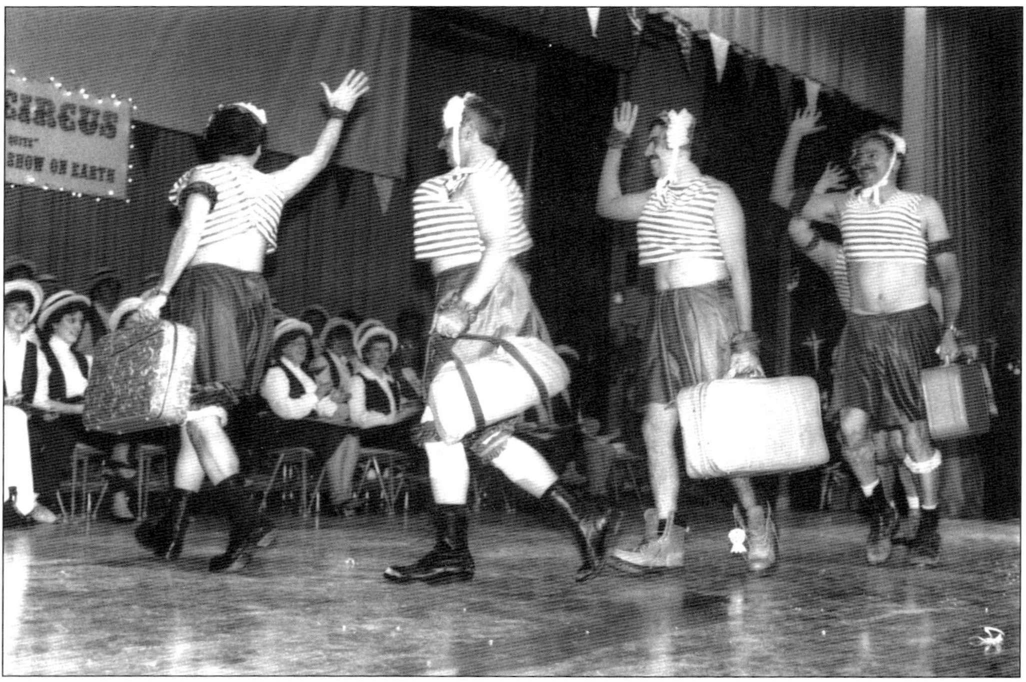

Another well-received group at the 1985 circus was the Clinical Q-Teez. Pictured are, from left to right, Dr. Charles Fedele, Dr. Robert Michaels, Dr. Joseph A. Scopelliti, and Dr. J. Thomas Danzi. Not visible is Dr. Kirk Tolhurst.

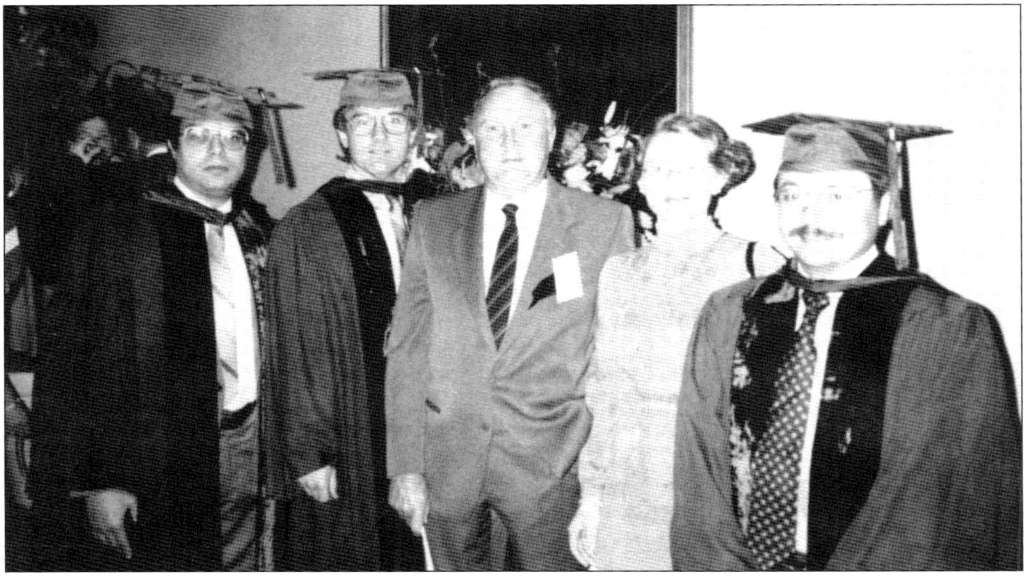

Clinic physicians inducted into the American College of Surgeons in 1986 include, from left to right, Dr. Alfredo Llinas, Dr. Stephen Annest, Dr. John Thomas, Dr. Irene Nasaduke, and Dr. Brian Charlton. Dr. Donald Guthrie was a founding member of the American College of Surgeons.

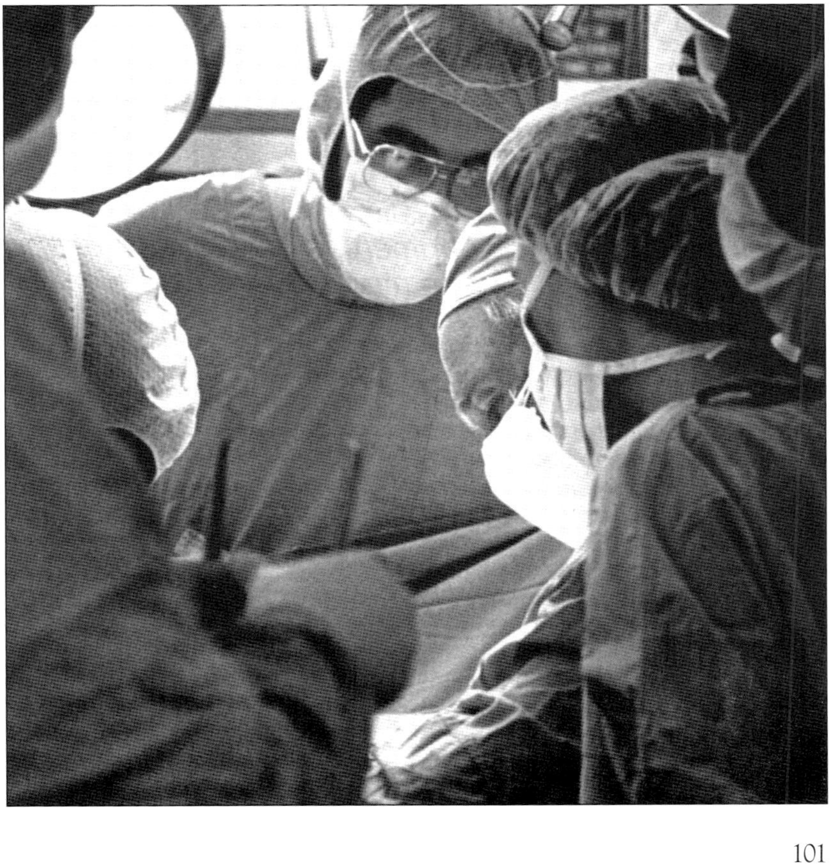

The vascular surgery team at Guthrie Clinic in the mid-1980s includes Dr. Stephen Annest, Dr. Narayan Deshmukh, and section chief Dr. John Thomas.

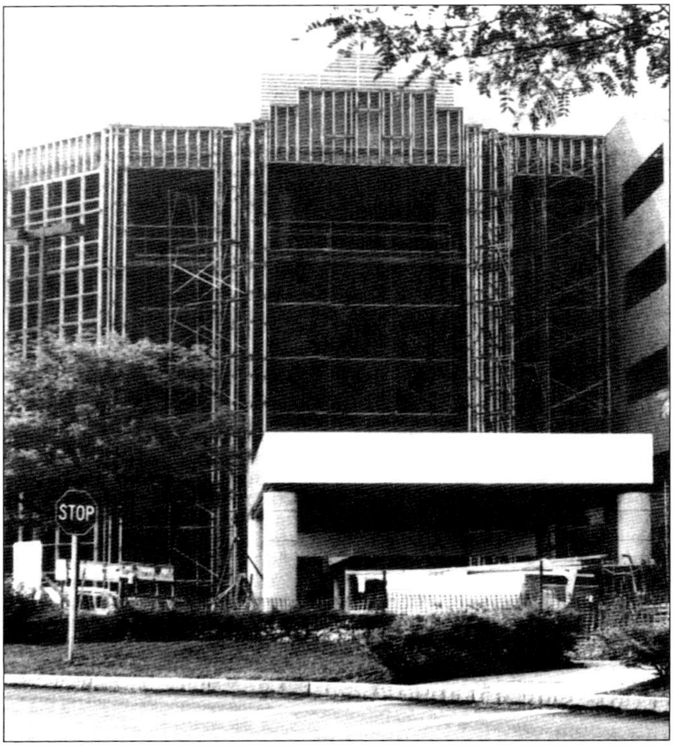

This photograph captures the clinic expansion mid-construction in the summer of 1988. The facility was a five-story, $10-million expansion.

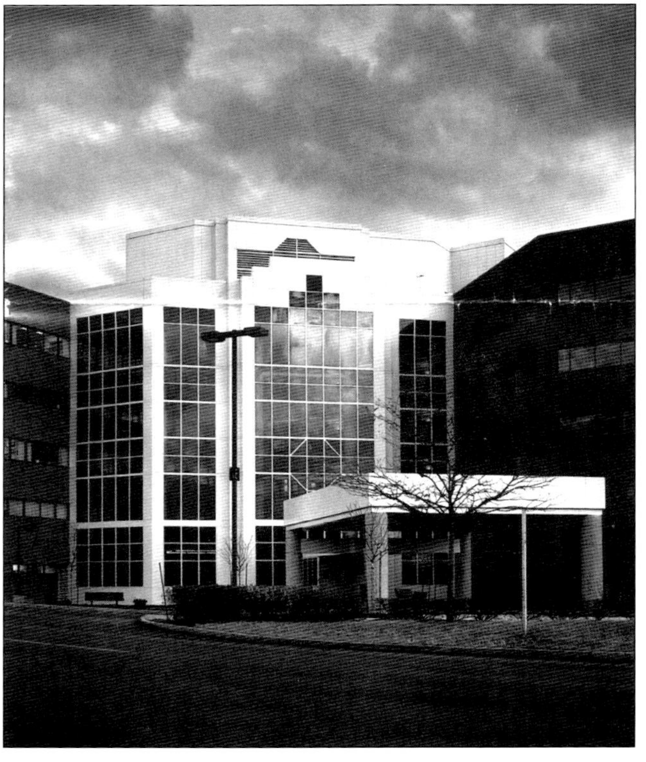

This picture shows a view of the completed facility (far right) and the new atrium connecting the two medical office buildings. Later the atrium was used as the primary entrance to both the clinic and hospital.

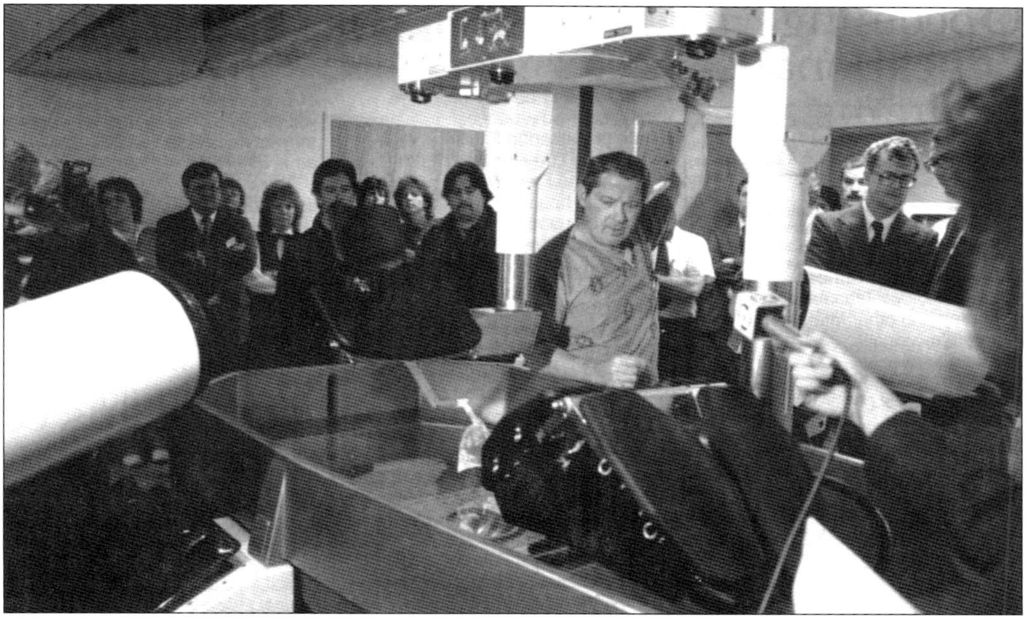

Always at the forefront with new technologies that benefited patients, shown here is the introduction of the lithotripter used to treat kidney stones.

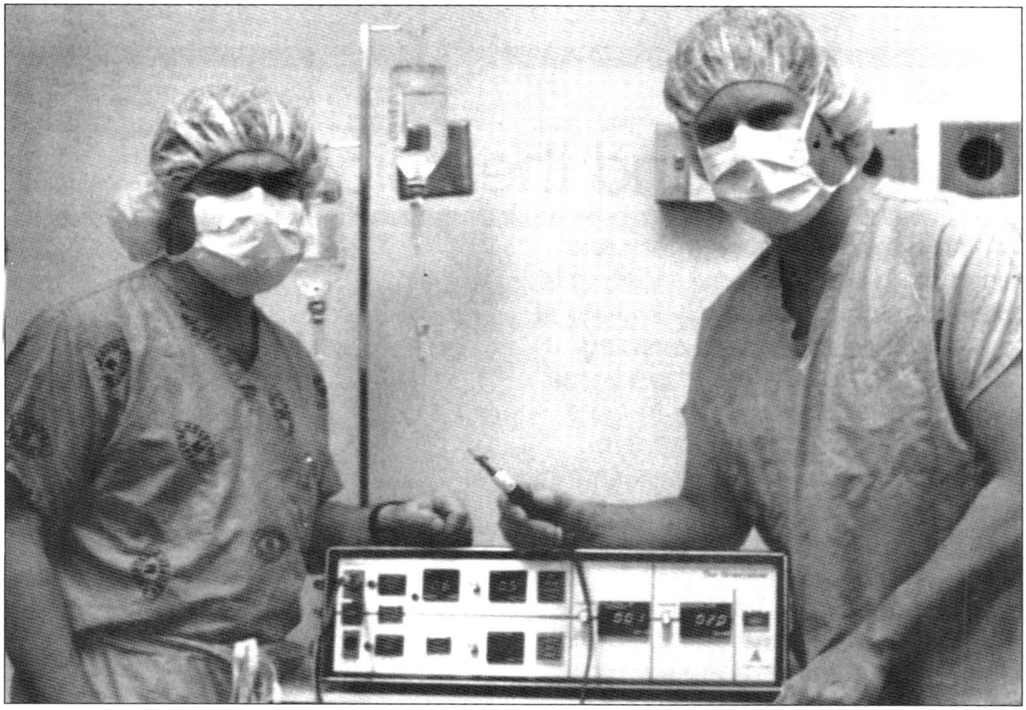

Dr. Terence Devine (right), chief of ophthalmology, poses with a new ocusystem at Guthrie Clinic—the only such device in the world at the time.

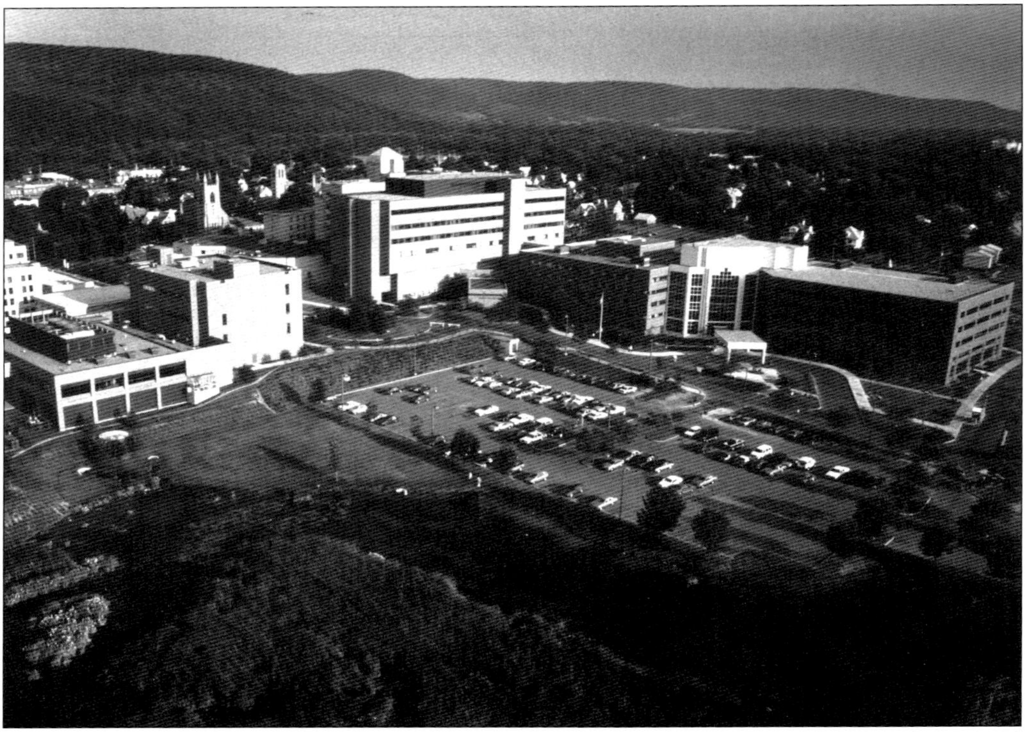

This photograph shows Guthrie Clinic's Sayre campus as it looked in 1989 after the second Guthrie Clinic building was opened.

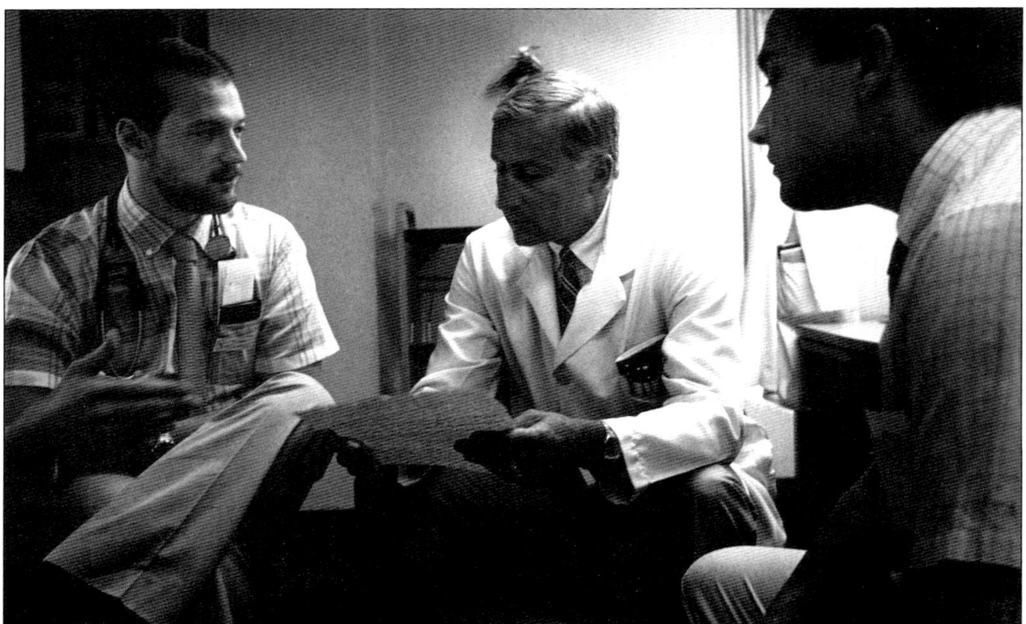

Dr. Mal Homan (left), endocrinology, and Dr. J. Thomas Danzi (center), gastroenterology, are shown with an unidentified resident (right) as they consult on a patient's care.

Nine

Meeting Community Needs

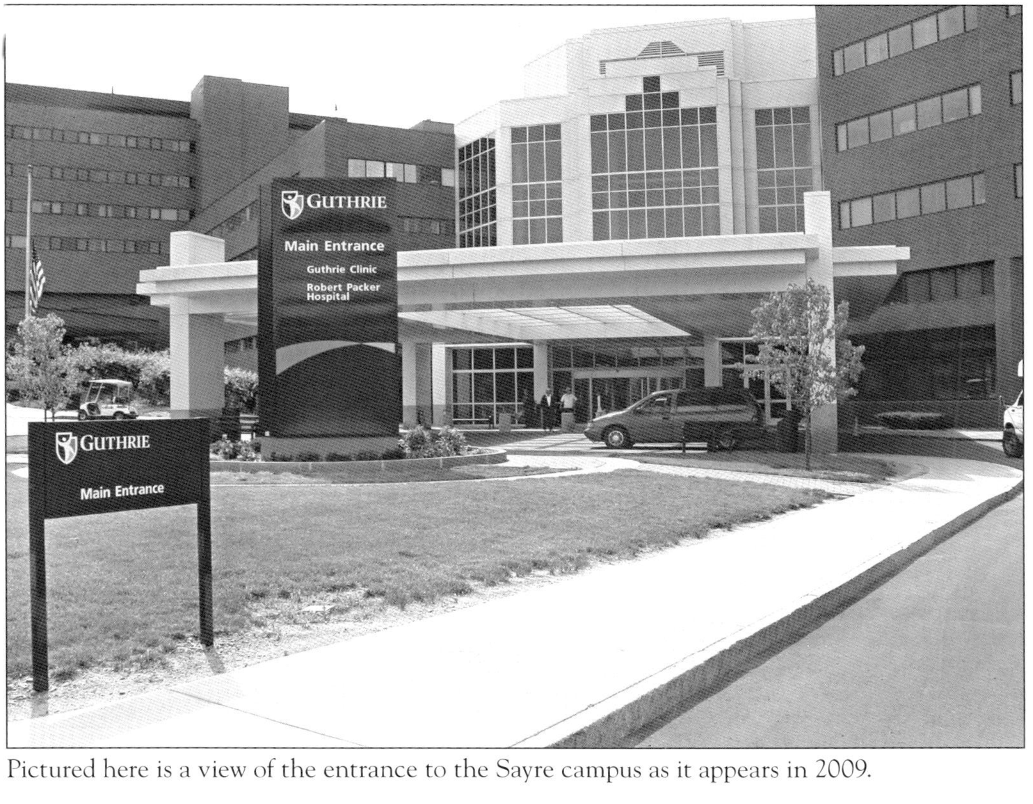

Pictured here is a view of the entrance to the Sayre campus as it appears in 2009.

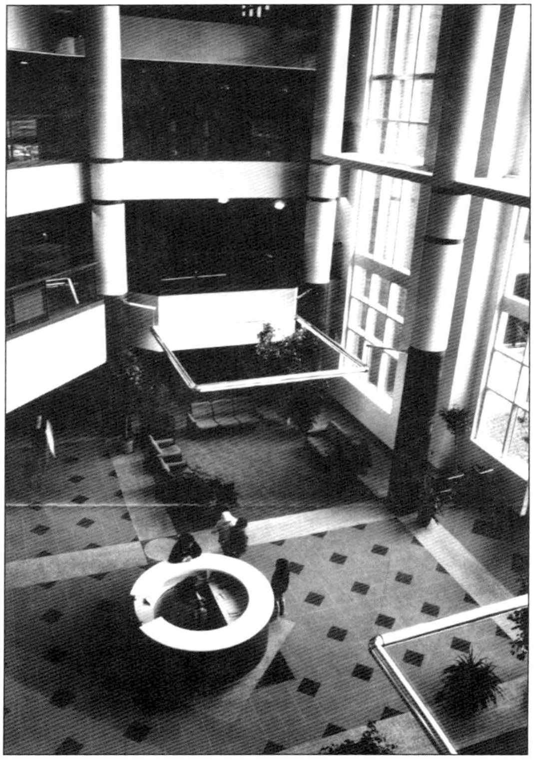

This photograph shows the clinic atrium as it appeared when the new building opened.

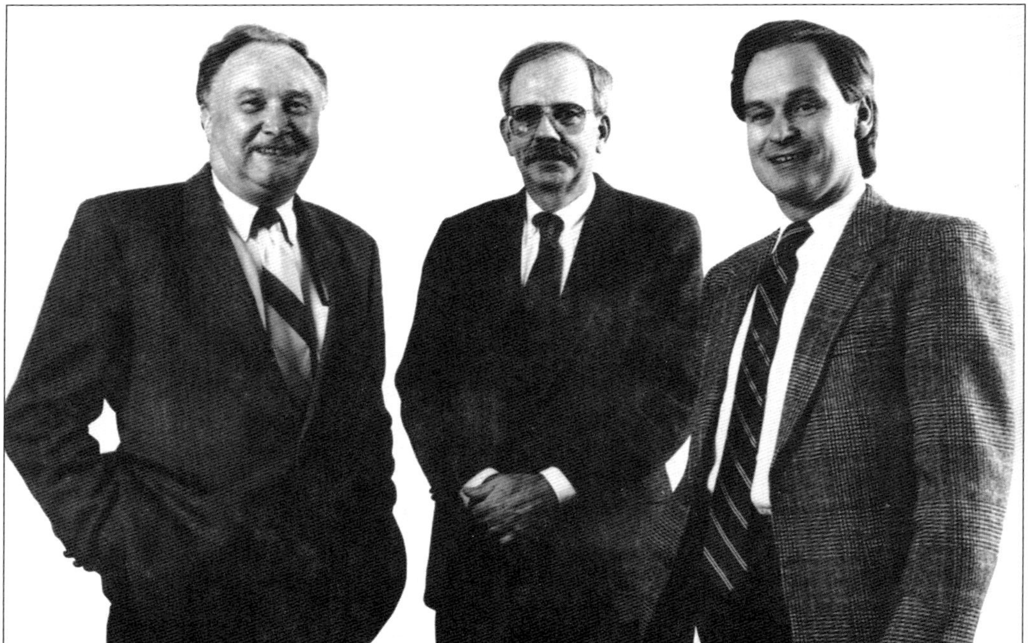

Guthrie Clinic and Guthrie Medical Center leadership in the early 1990s includes, from left to right, Dr. John Thomas, Ralph Meyer, and Dr. Blaine Cobb.

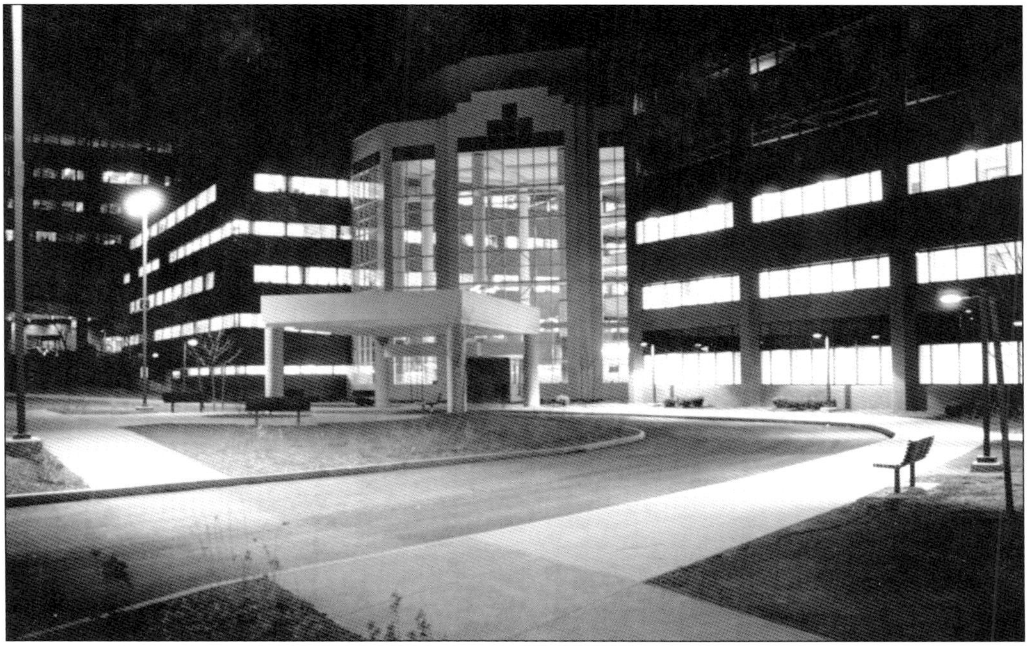

This exterior evening view shows how the atrium (center) connects the clinic buildings (shown on each side of the atrium). Inside the atrium, crosswalks provide passage between each floor of the clinic's two buildings.

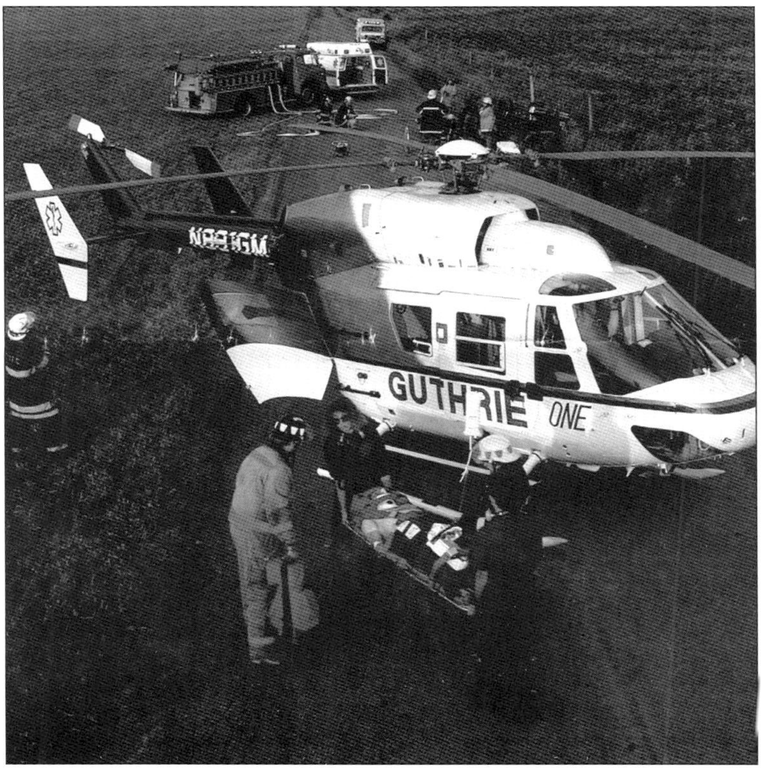

The health care system has evolved from the use of a horse-drawn ambulance to a medical helicopter program that began in 1989, yet another sign of how health care has advanced during the past century.

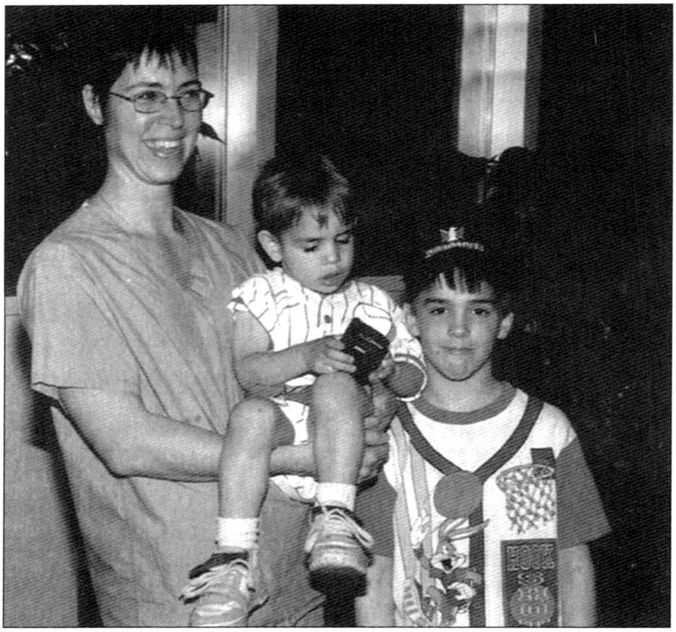

Cardiac surgeon Dr. Felice Reitknecht shares a happy moment holding a recovered Trevor Belcher as his brother, Tyler, stands nearby. Trevor became a local celebrity after Dr. Reitknecht and her surgical team saved his life in a dramatic fashion by reviving the boy when he suffered from severe hypothermia.

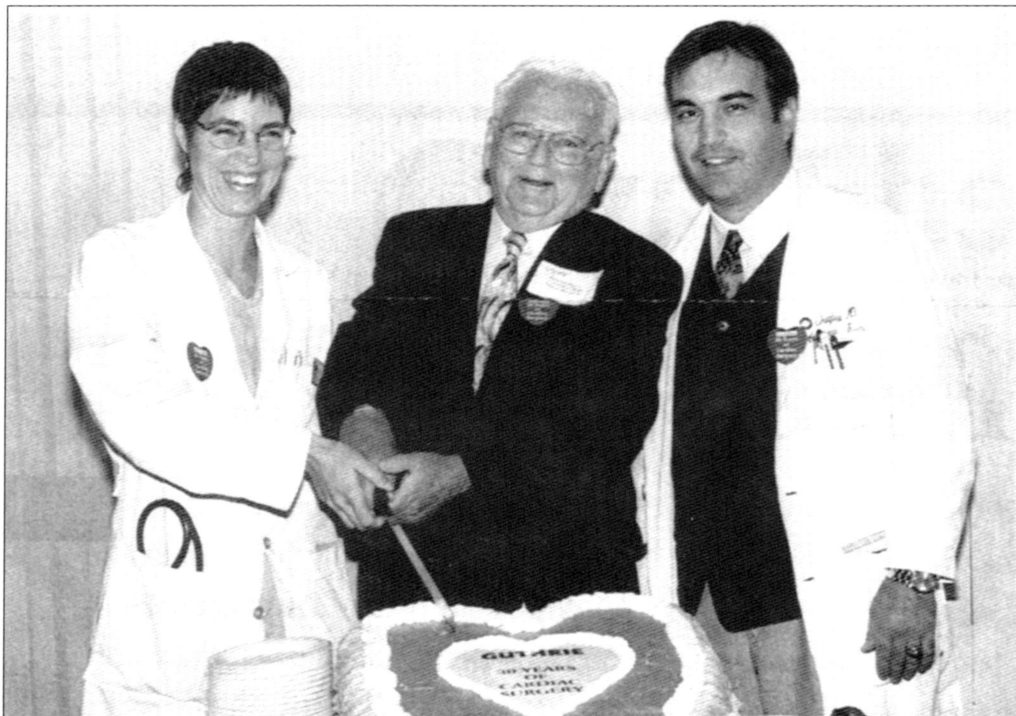

Physicians, clinical staff, and patients celebrated 30 years of cardiac surgery at Guthrie Clinic and Robert Packer Hospital during an event held in November 1996. From left to right, Dr. Felice Reitknecht, Dick Hogan (a former patient and founding member of the Pedigraft Club), and Dr. Robert Quigley prepare to cut into a heart-shaped cake.

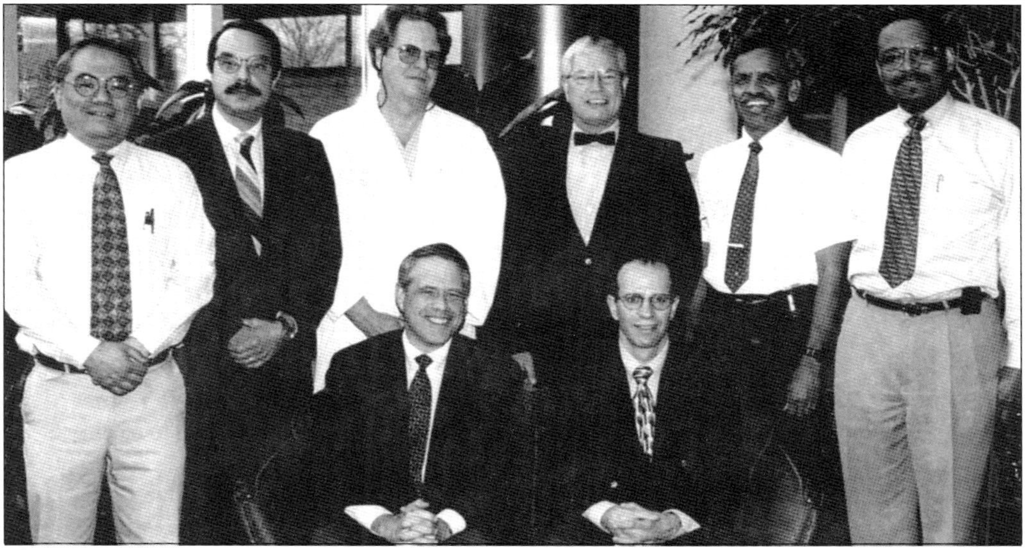

The members of the Guthrie Clinic Board of Directors in 1999 are, from left to right, (first row) Dr. Kevin V. Carey and Dr. Robert E. Cohen; (second row) Mei-Chang Cheng, Alfredo Llinas, Terence Devine, Edward J. Jones, Narayan Deshmukh, and Dr. Ferrol J. Lee.

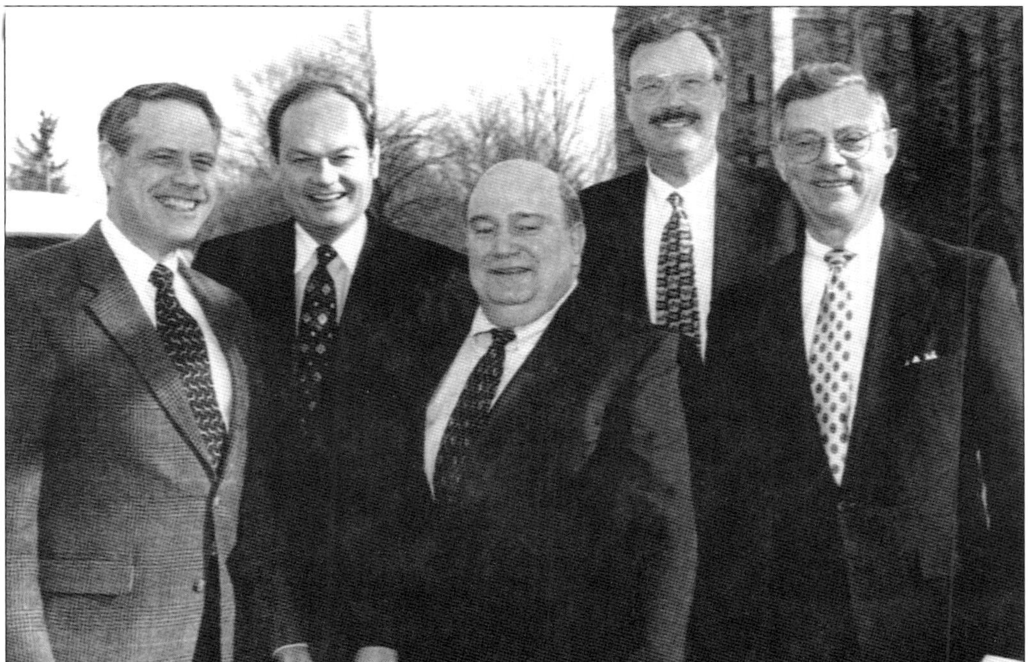

Corning Hospital joined Guthrie Healthcare System in 1999. Representing the boards of directors who endorsed the relationship are, from left to right, Dr. Kevin V. Carey, Guthrie Clinic president and chief executive officer; Mark Stensager, Guthrie Healthcare System chief executive officer; John Pignatore, Corning Hospital chief executive officer; William H. Ransom III, chairman Guthrie Healthcare System board; and Stephen L. Albertalli, president, Corning Hospital board.

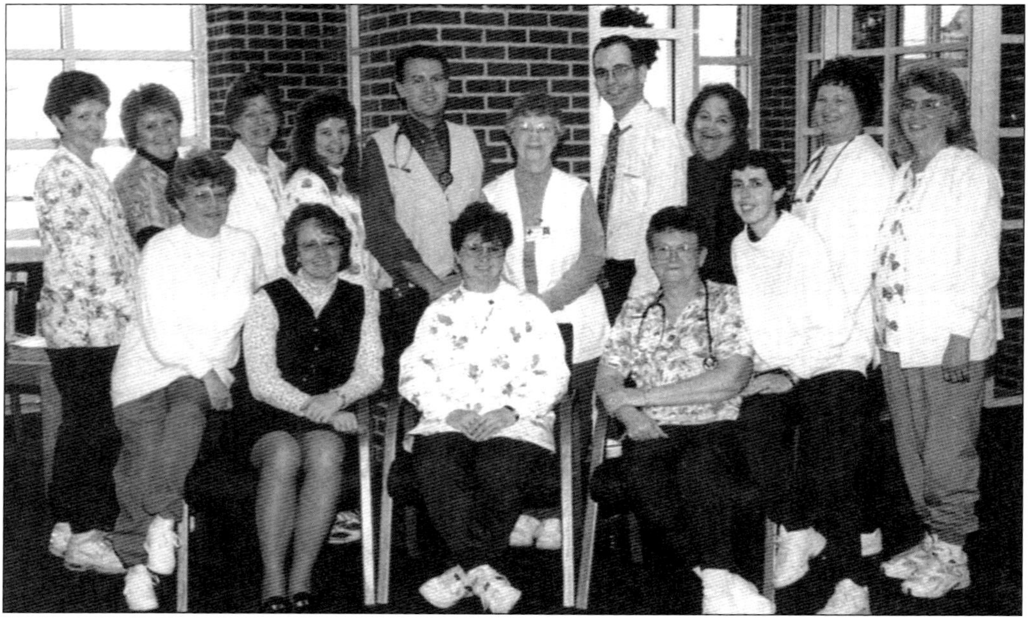

The clinic's regional office network makes local access to high-quality care available in communities in New York and Pennsylvania. Pictured here are members of the Wellsboro regional office staff who opened a new office location in 1999.

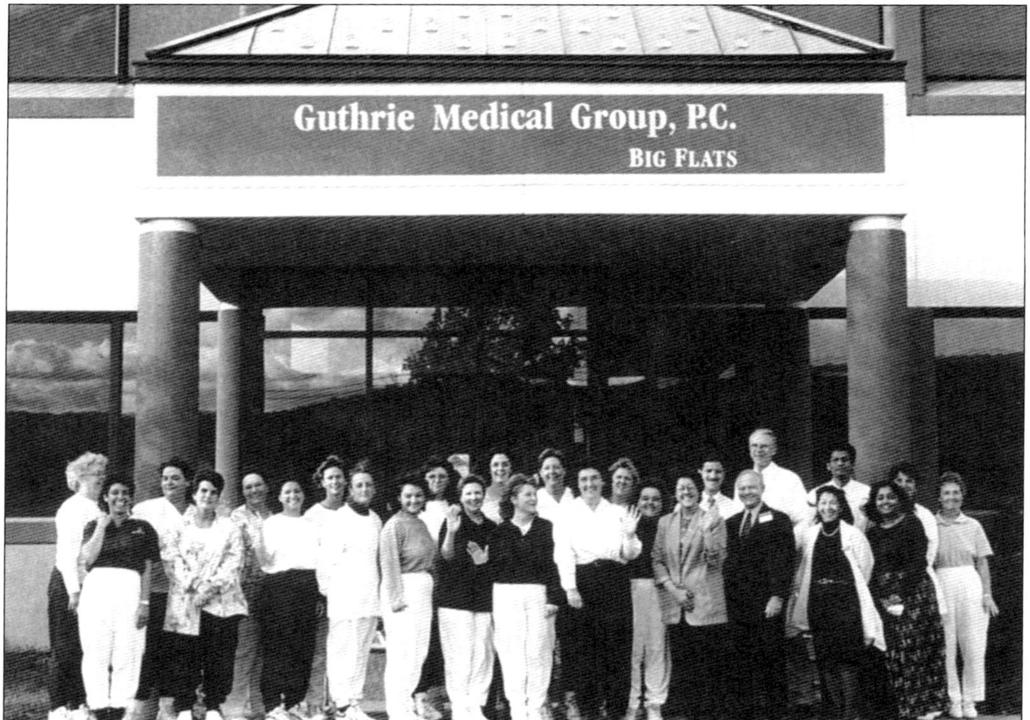

The physicians and staff of the Big Flats regional office pose in front of their new location in the fall of 1999.

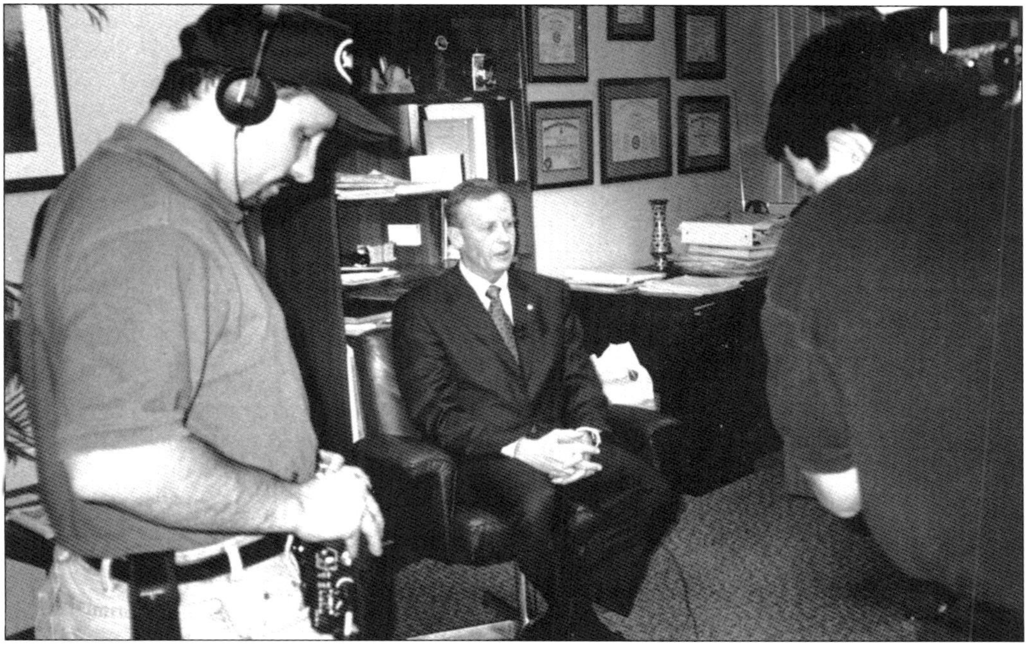

Cardiologist Dr. Lynn A. Smaha was named president of the American Heart Association in the summer of 1999. At the time, Dr. Smaha served the clinic as its executive vice president.

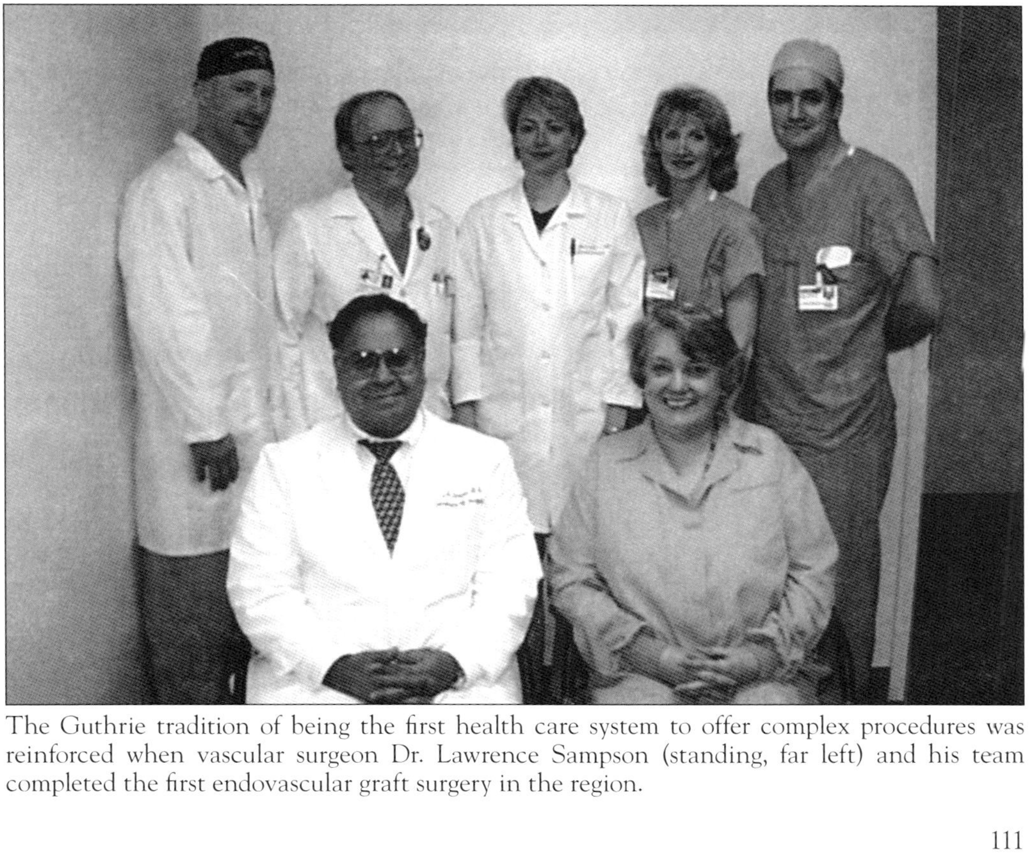

The Guthrie tradition of being the first health care system to offer complex procedures was reinforced when vascular surgeon Dr. Lawrence Sampson (standing, far left) and his team completed the first endovascular graft surgery in the region.

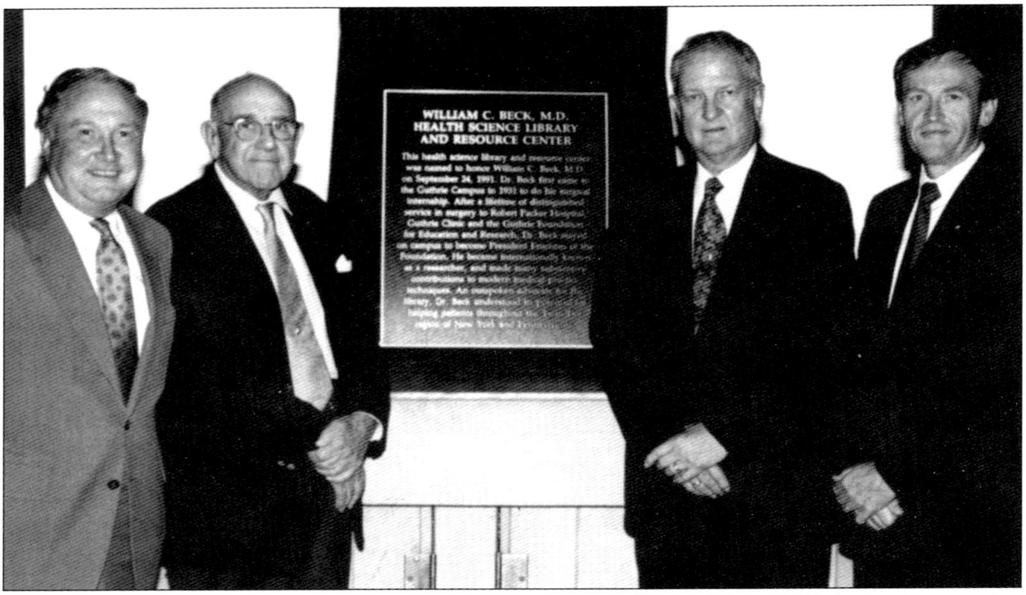

This picture, taken in 1992, shows Dr. William C. Beck (second from left) being honored as the health care system's medical library is dedicated in his name. Pictured from left to right are Dr. John Thomas, Dr. Beck, Robert Landy, and Dr. Lynn A. Smaha.

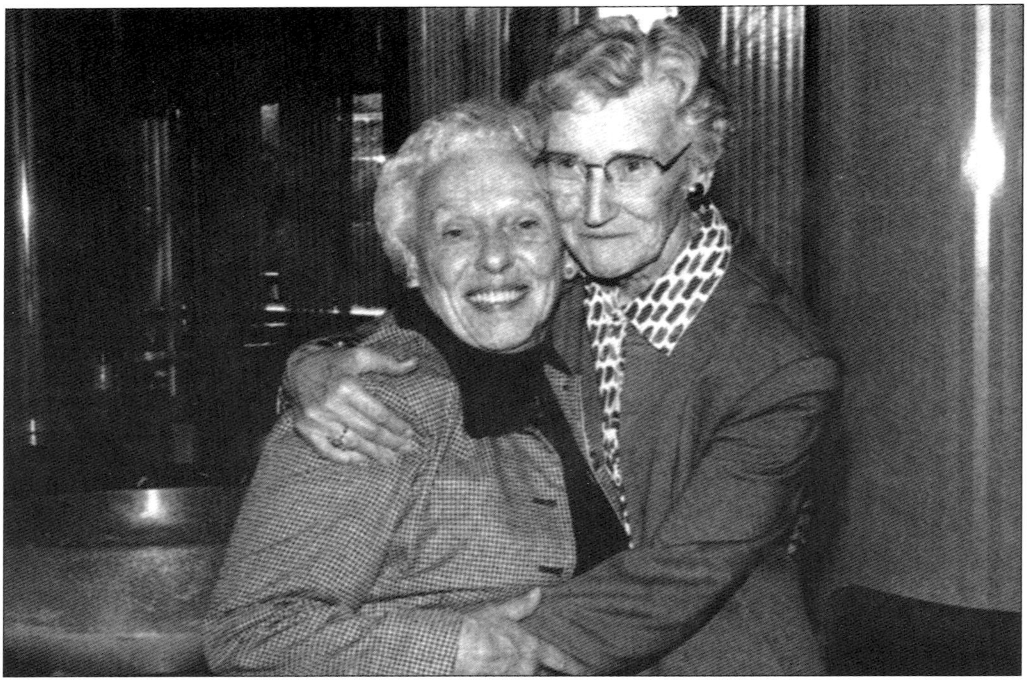

Jean Antes (right) was honored at her retirement after serving Guthrie Clinic for 27 years as the medical reference librarian. Antes created the circuit library program that serves a number of other smaller hospitals, providing them with up-to-date literature on a variety of medical topics. With her is longtime friend Beryl Cleary, graduate and retired faculty of the school of nursing and volunteer archivist.

Ten

THE NEW MILLENNIUM

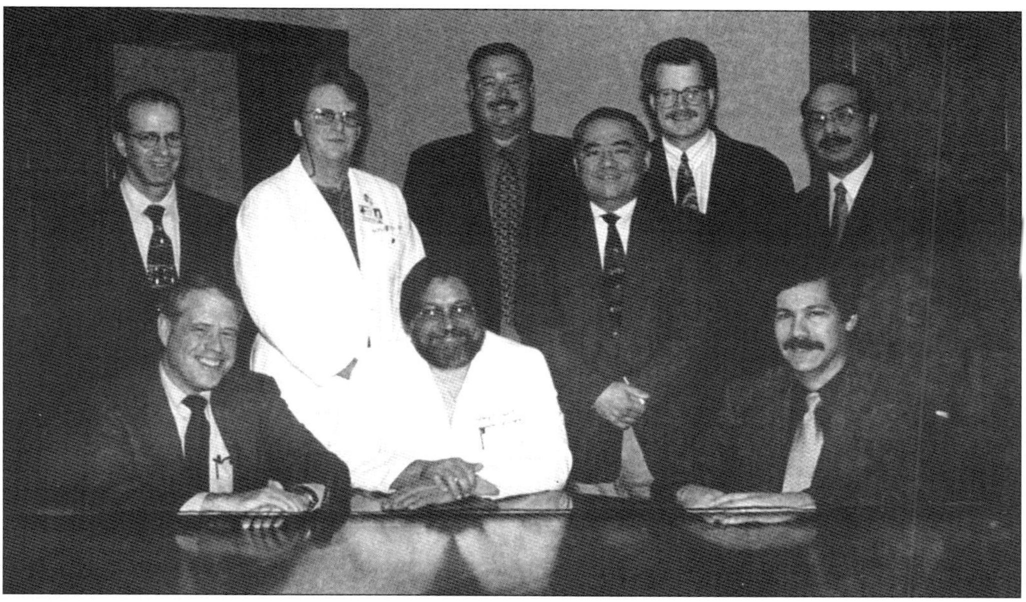

Guthrie Healthcare System board chairman William H. Ransom III (standing, center) met with the Guthrie Clinic Board of Directors as elected in 2000. Board members are, from left to right, (first row) Dr. Kevin V. Carey, Dr. Anthony Gillott, and Dr. Daniel Sporn; (second row) Dr. Robert E. Cohen, Dr. Terence Devine, Ransom, Dr. Mei-Chang Cheng, Dr. Thomas McDonald, and Dr. Alfredo Llinas.

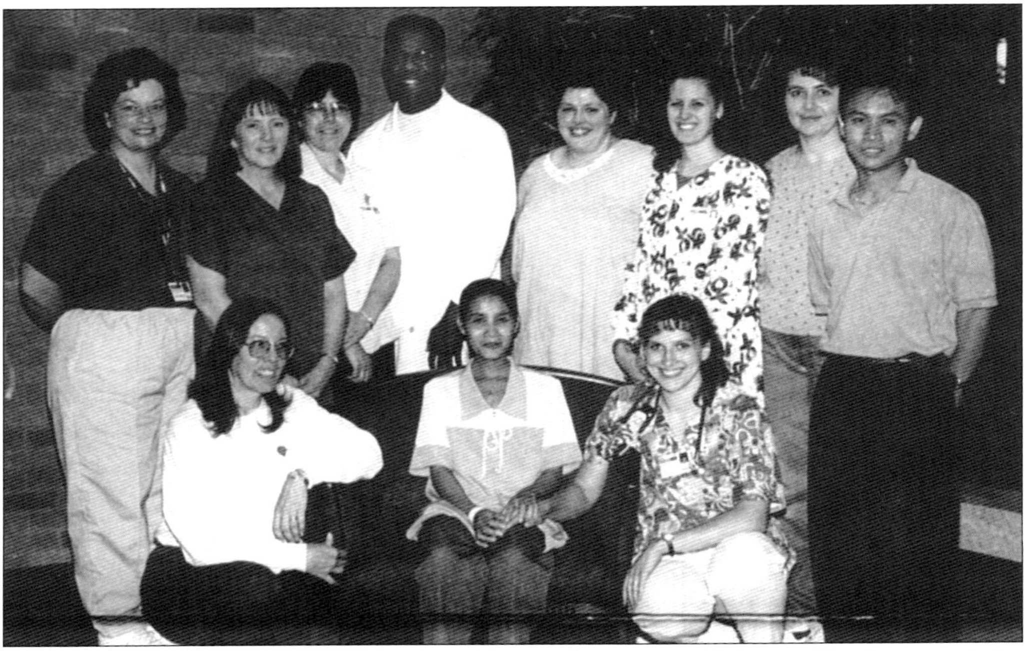

Dr. Nche Zama (white coat, back row) and hospital nursing staff from 6 Northwest and the intensive care unit (ICU) wish Lek Yea (seated) well as she prepares to be discharged. Yea, a Cambodian woman, came to the hospital under the auspices of the International Heart to Heart Foundation. Dr. Zama and the staff cared for her during her stay.

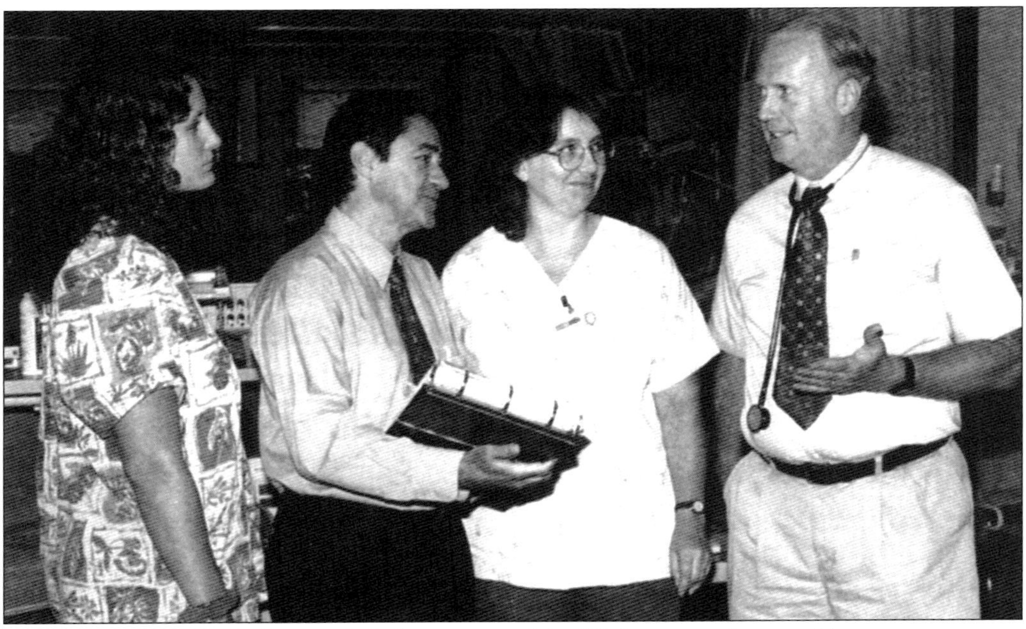

In 2000, nurses from the hospital's dialysis unit and the ICU partnered to provide a new treatment option called continuous renal replacement therapy (CRRT) to ICU patients. Discussing CRRT are, from left to right, Shiela Groover, RN, dialysis; Dr. Felix DeSio, nephrology; Vicki Haiges, RN, 2ICU (2nd level ICU); and Dr. William Cady, chief of nephrology.

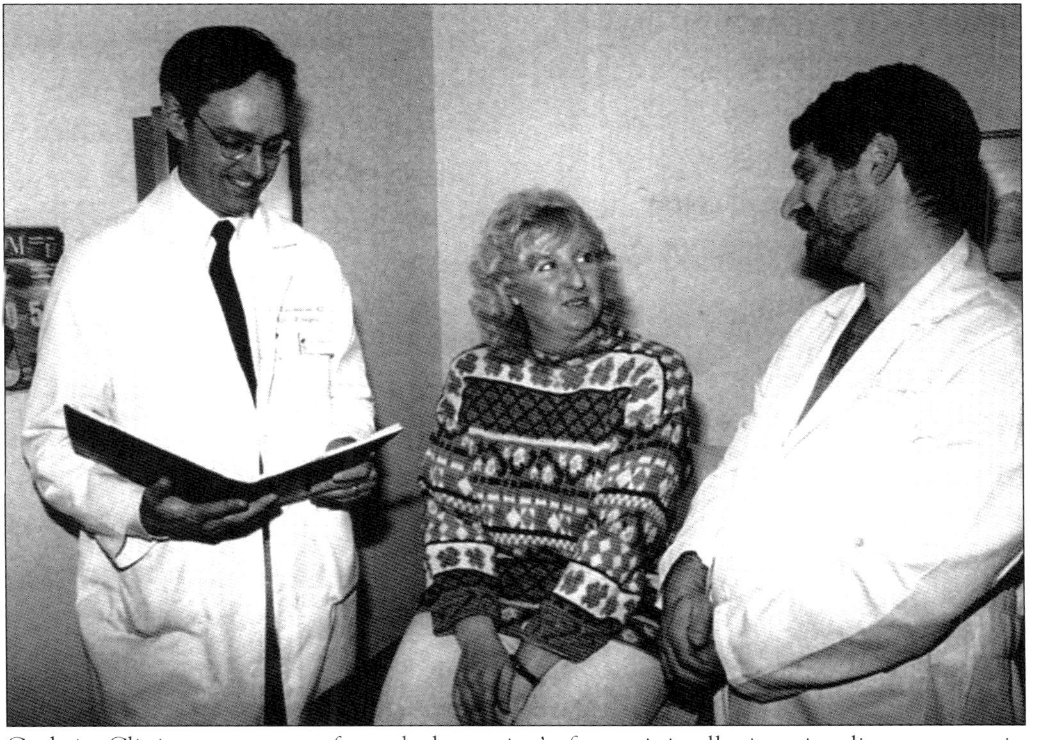

Guthrie Clinic surgeons performed the region's first minimally invasive liver surgery in December 2000. Dr. Thomas VanderMeer (left) and Dr. Steven Simon (right) discuss Roberta Bull's (center) recovery.

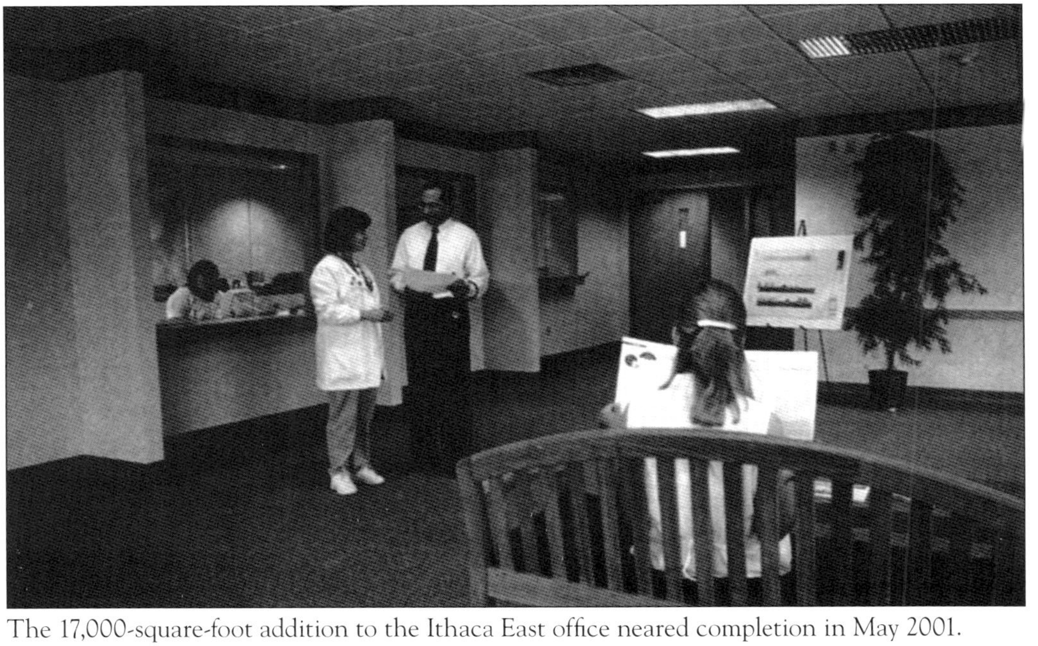

The 17,000-square-foot addition to the Ithaca East office neared completion in May 2001.

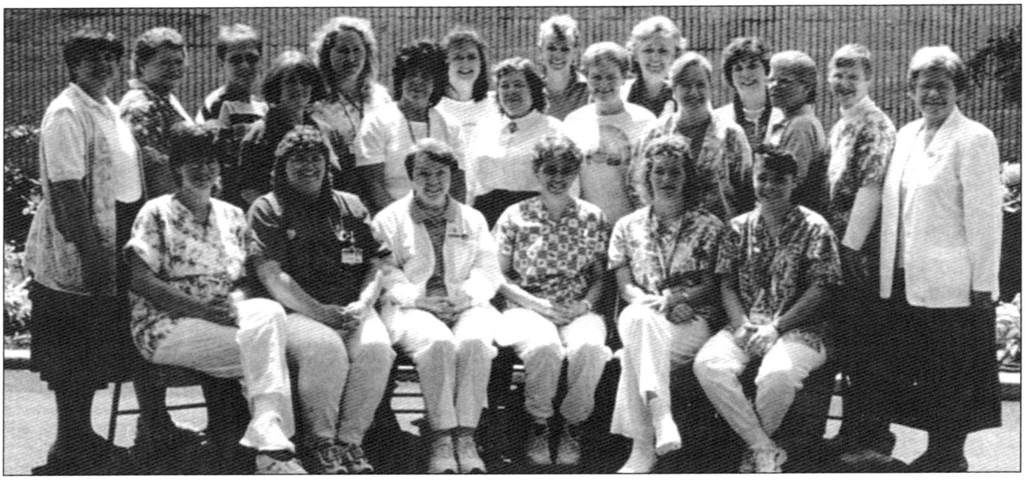

Guthrie Healthcare System's Troy Community Hospital was recognized in June 2001 as one of the top four hospitals in the nation for nursing satisfaction. Assembled in this photograph is a group of nurses working at the hospital at that time.

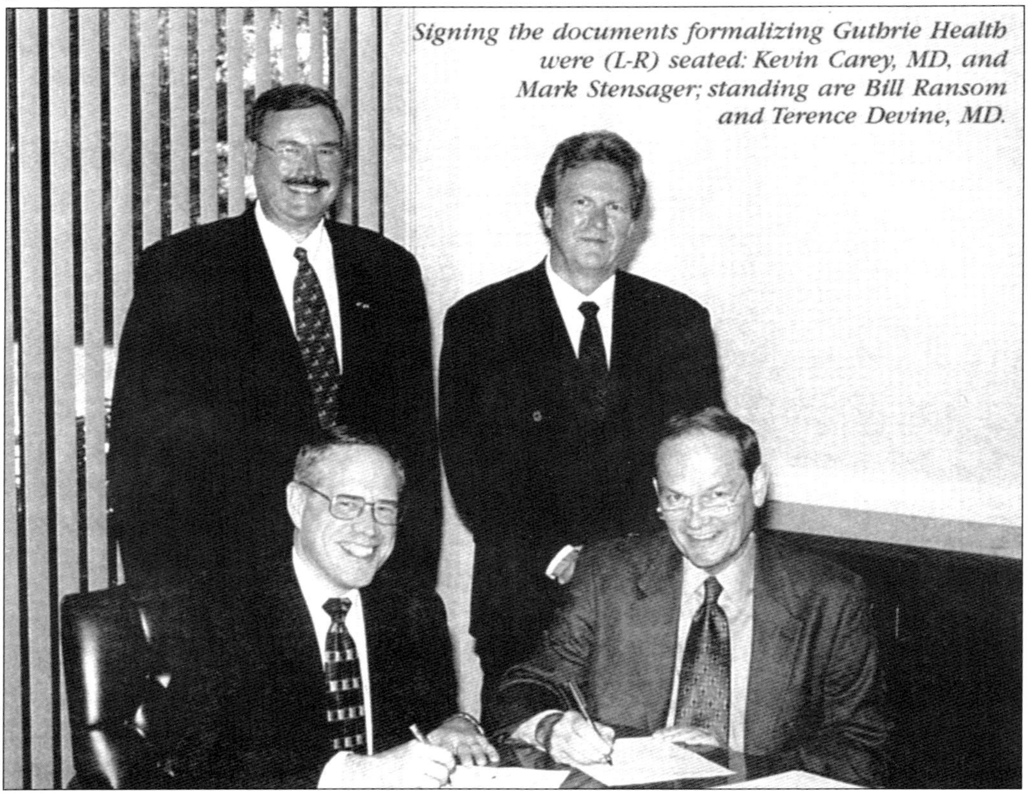
Signing the documents formalizing Guthrie Health
were (L-R) seated: Kevin Carey, MD, and
Mark Stensager; standing are Bill Ransom
and Terence Devine, MD.

Created by Guthrie Clinic and Guthrie Healthcare System, Guthrie Health became a reality on June 13, 2001. Pictured here are, from left to right, (first row) Guthrie Clinic president and chief executive officer Dr. Kevin V. Carey and Guthrie Healthcare System president and chief executive officer Mark Stensager; (second row) Guthrie Healthcare System board chairman William H. Ransom III and Guthrie Clinic board chairman Dr. Terence Devine.

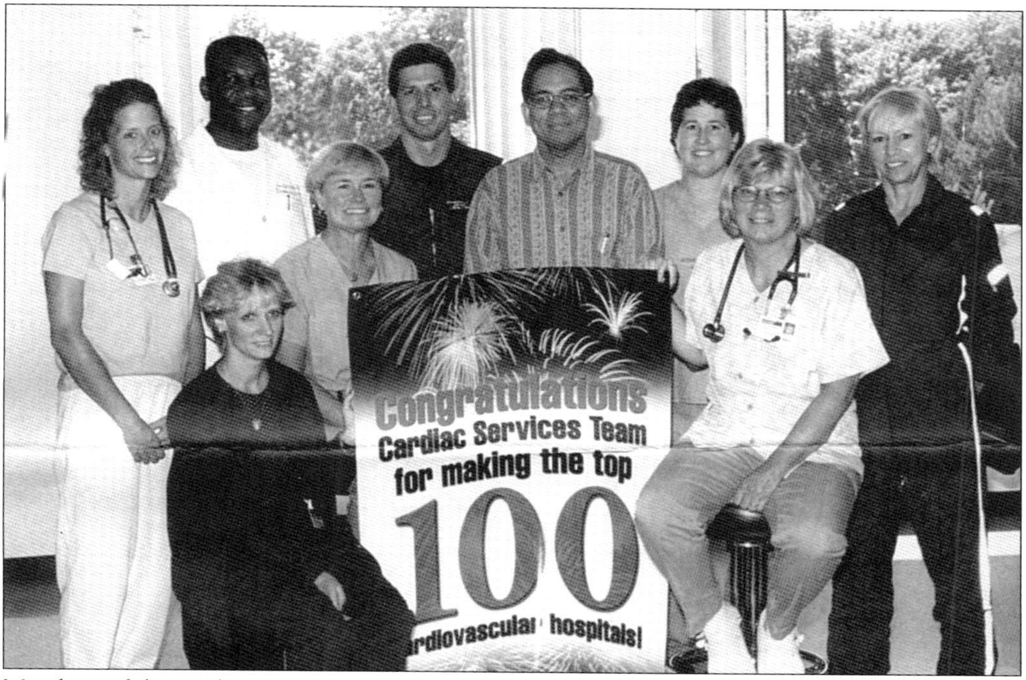
Congratulations
Cardiac Services Team
for making the top
100
rdiovascular hospitals!

Members of the cardiac care team celebrate Robert Packer Hospital being named to the 100 top cardiovascular hospitals list for the first time in 2001.

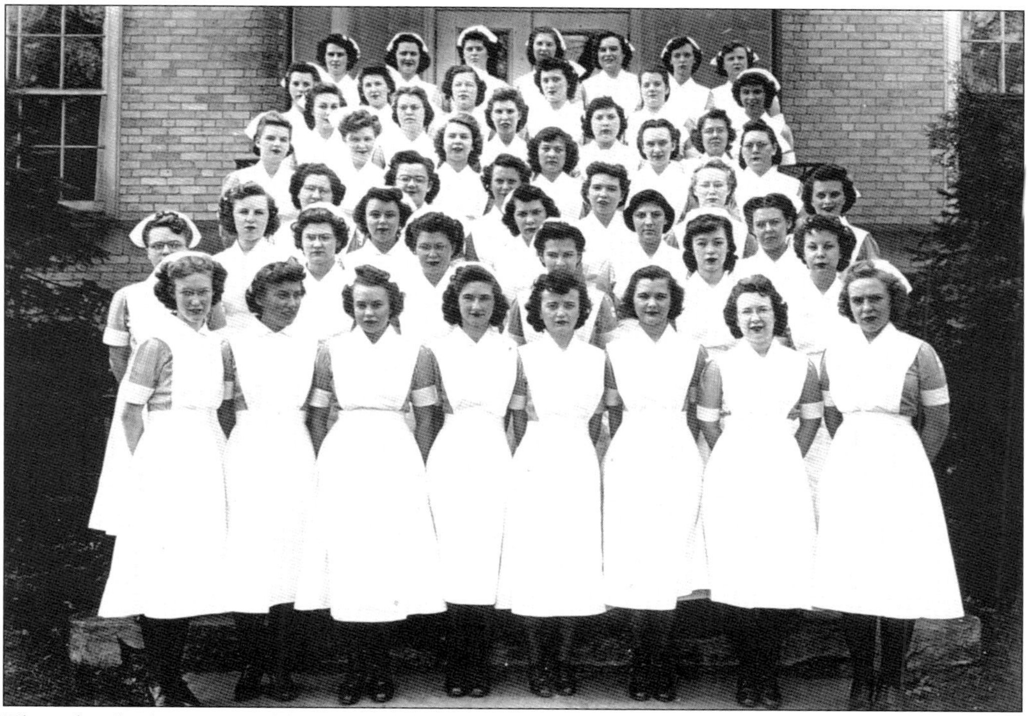

The school of nursing celebrated 100 years of excellence in nursing in 2001. Shown here is one of the largest classes to graduate from the program, the class of 1947.

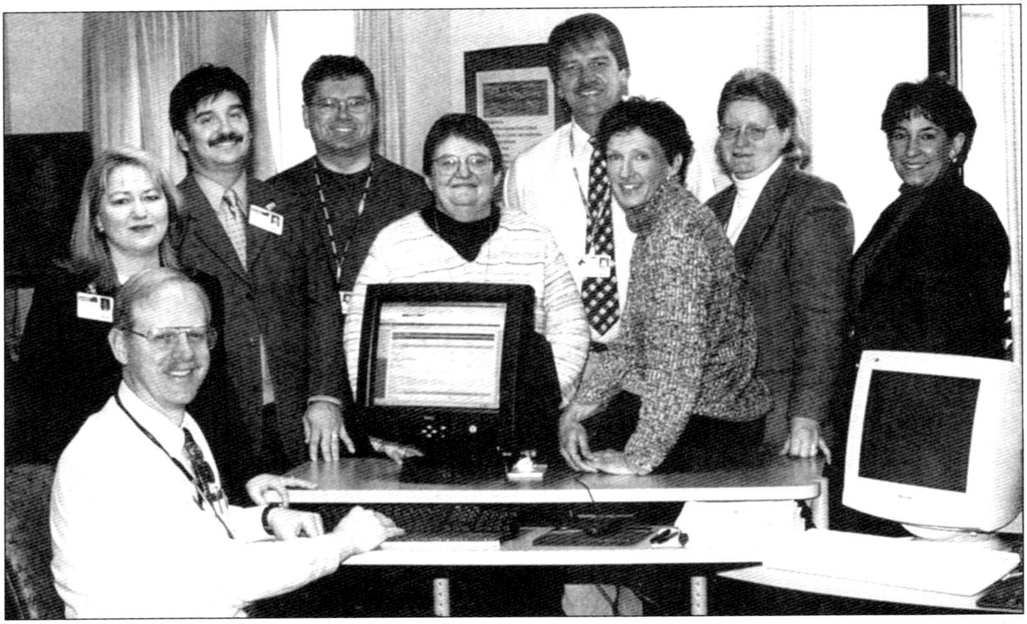

Electronic medical records debut at Guthrie Health in 2002. Pictured here from left to right are members of the Epic implementation team: Dr. Thomas A. Yaeger, chief information officer Mary Mannix, information services vice president Dale Swingle, Craig Wilhelm, Maria Worden, Robert Gould, Susan Fogel, Christine Personius, and Jackie Phillips.

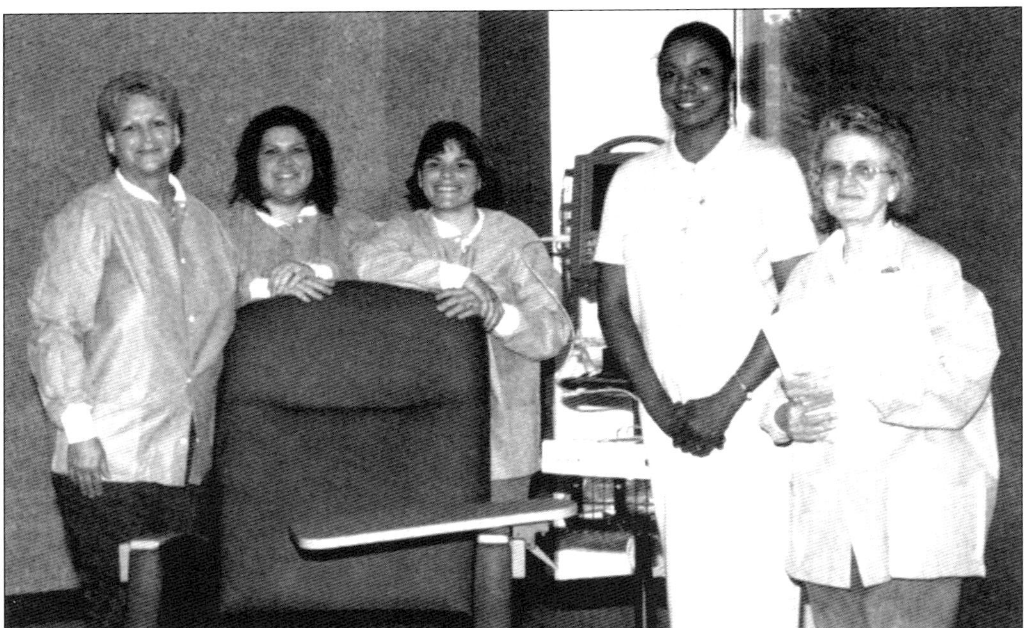

To meet the growing demand for same-day procedures, in 2002 Guthrie Healthcare System opened a same-day surgery center, located on the second floor of the Big Flats regional office. Here staff gathers in one of the preparation and recovery bays at the center.

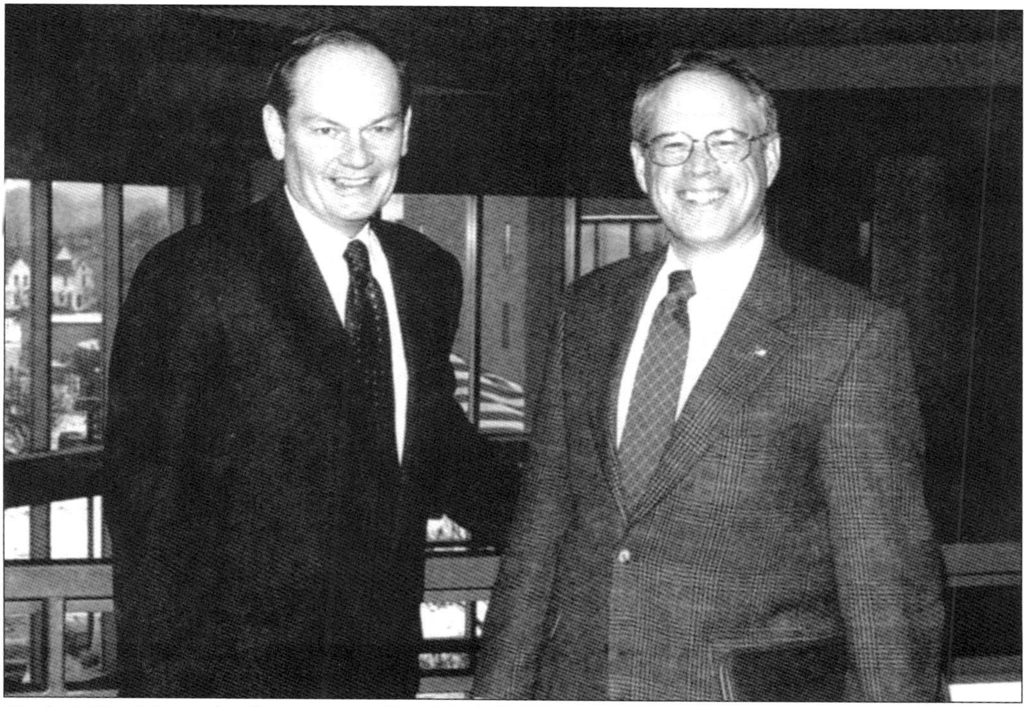
Guthrie Health co-chief executive officer Mark Stensager (left), administrative affairs, and Guthrie Health co-chief executive officer Dr. Kevin V. Carey, medical affairs, worked collaboratively to set the course for the new organization.

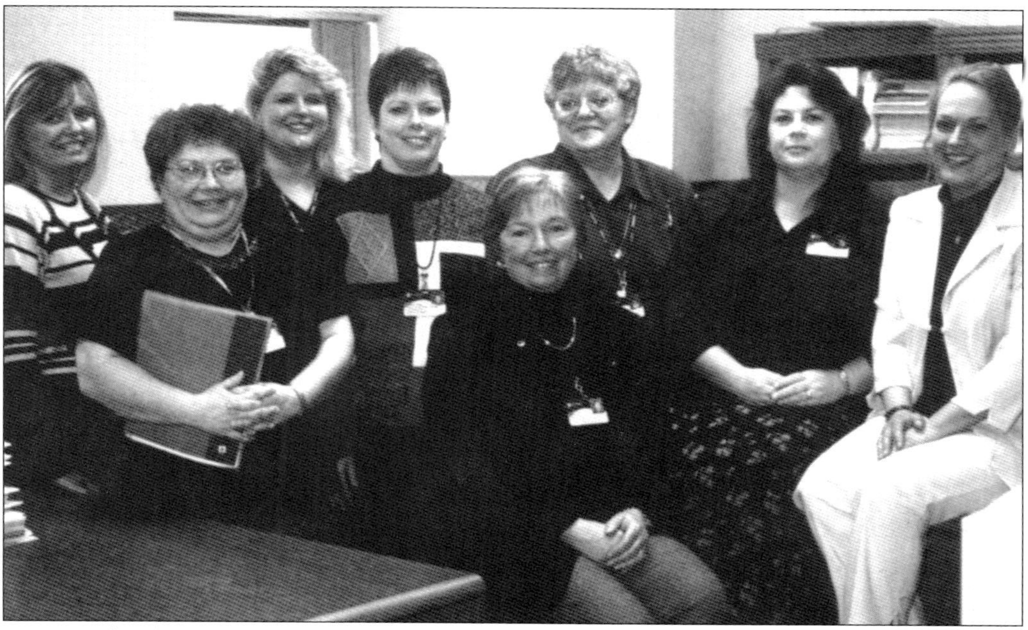
In 2003, the clinical research department staff supported 120 clinical trials. Some of the team is shown here. From left to right are Kami Hoey, Susan Hadlock, Deb Shady, Shelley Jones, Elaine Wall, Sue Para, Deb Sugg, and Michelle Cianfoni.

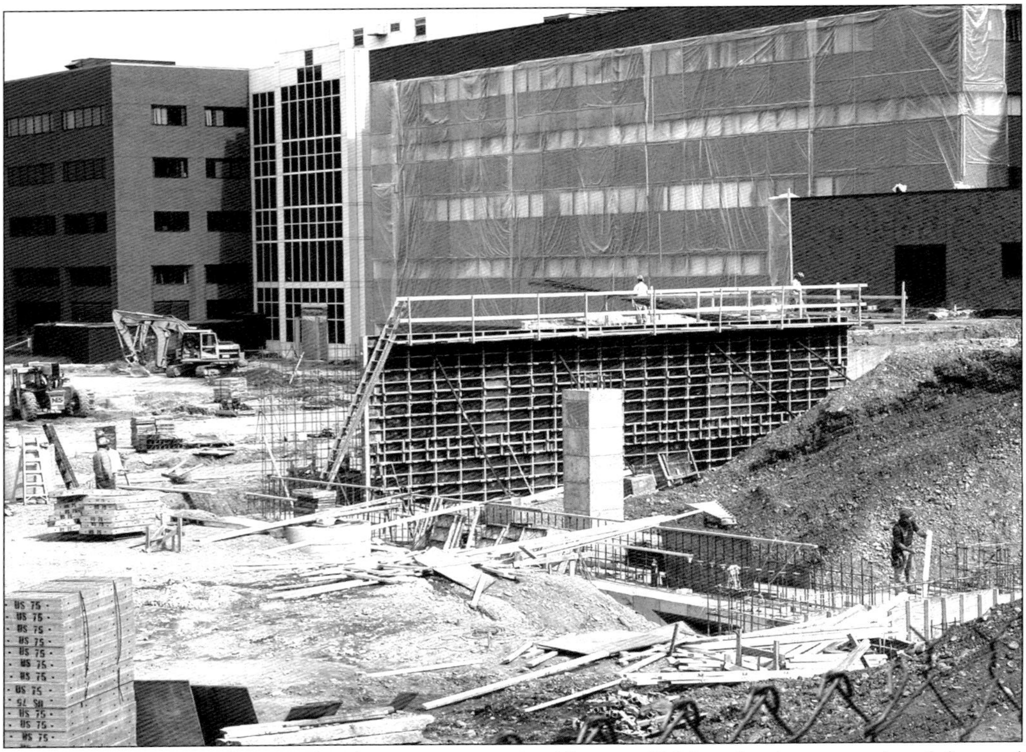

Construction got under way for the new surgery building in 2004 and, when completed, housed the most advanced, state-of-the-art surgical suites in the region.

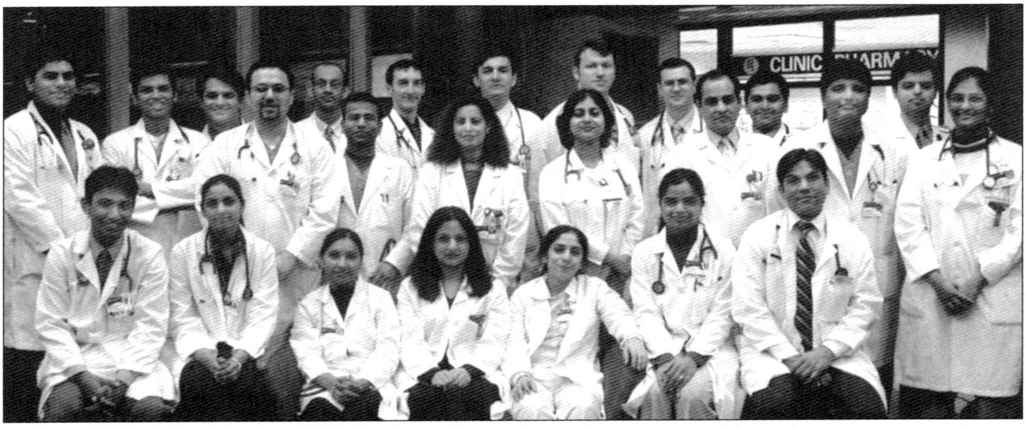

One of the fundamental principles brought to Sayre by Dr. Donald Guthrie was the value of medical education to patient care. In 2005, Robert Packer Hospital internal medicine residents (pictured) scored the second-highest score in the nation on the in-training exam.

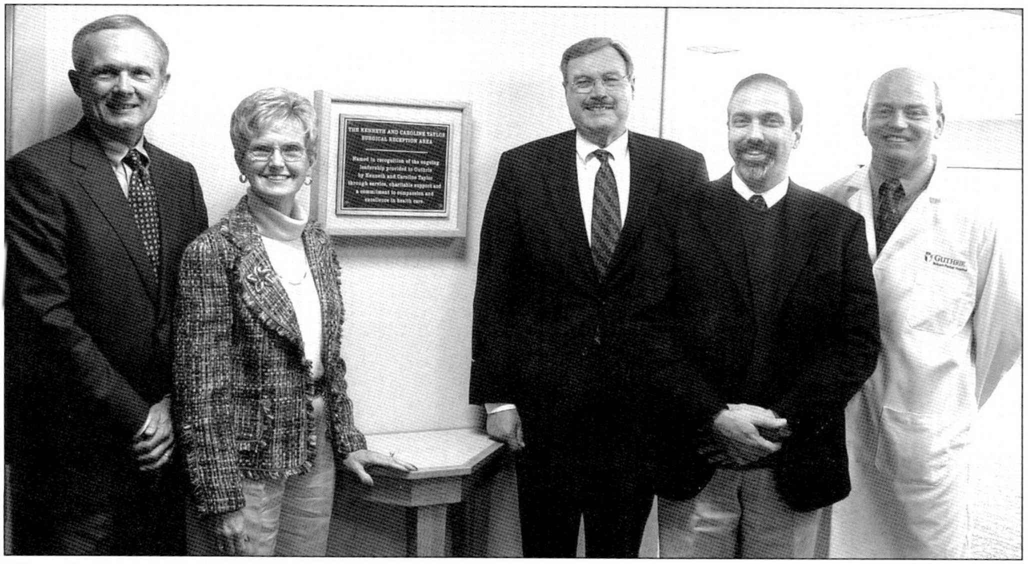

The dedication of the Kenneth and Caroline Taylor Surgical Reception Area was held December 12, 2005, in honor of the Taylors' $1-million gift to Building the Future…the Campaign for Guthrie Health. Shown here from left to right are Kenneth Taylor, Caroline Taylor, Guthrie Healthcare System Board chairman William H. Ransom III, clinic president Dr. Joseph Scopelliti, and chief of anesthesiology Dr. Daniel Brown.

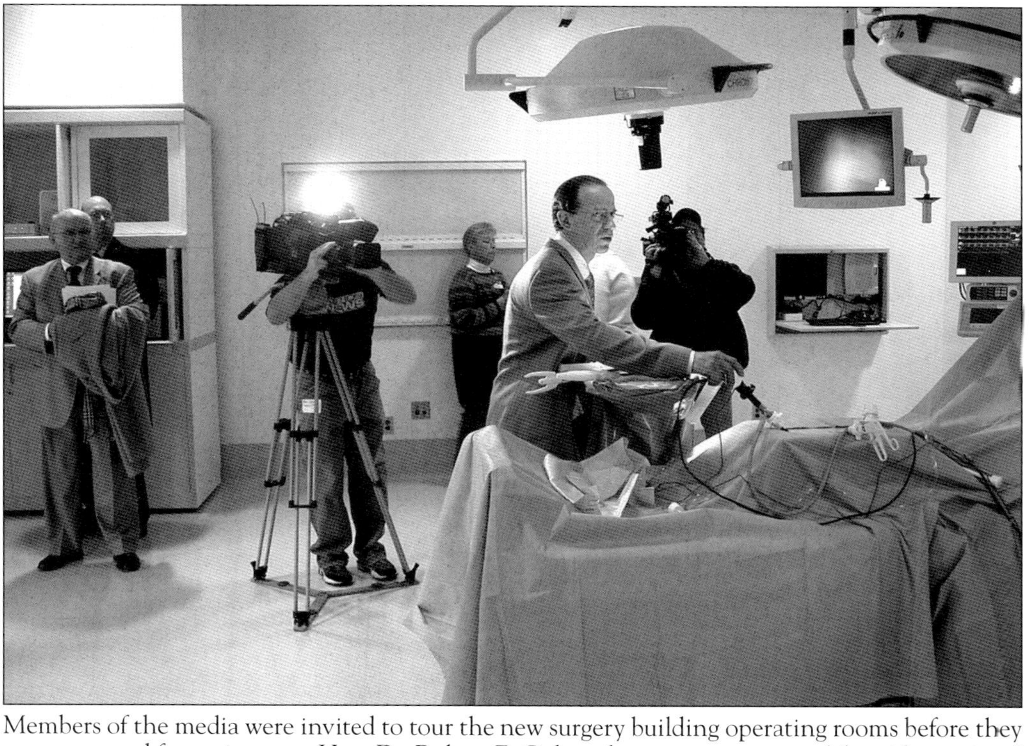

Members of the media were invited to tour the new surgery building operating rooms before they were prepared for patient use. Here Dr. Robert E. Cohen demonstrates some of the video-assisted capabilities of one of the new rooms to regional media.

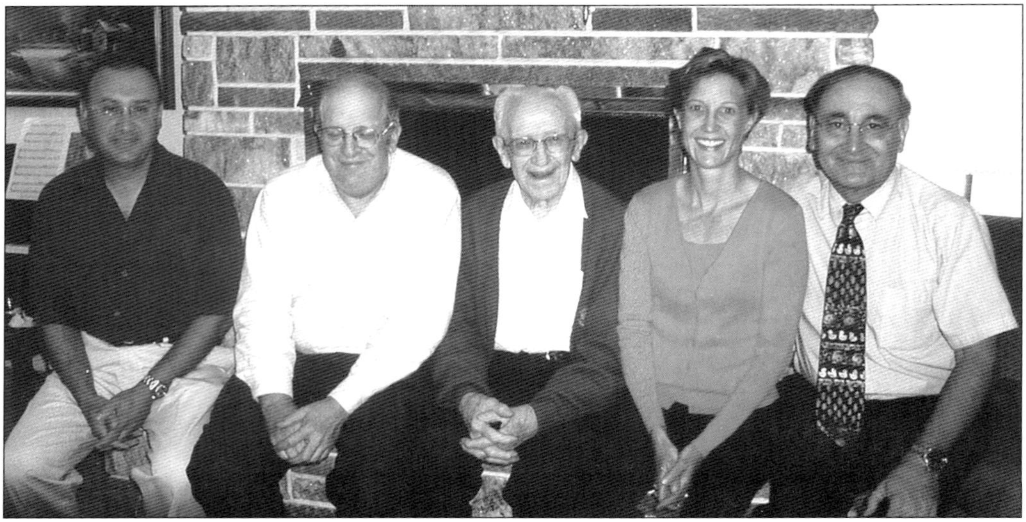

Helping to celebrate the 95th birthday of Dr. James Flood, one of Guthrie Clinic's previous generations of physicians who joined in 1946, are fellow dermatologists. Pictured are, from left to right, Dr. Richard Martines, Dr. Henry Shenfield, Dr. Flood, Dr. Kimberly Silvers, and Dr. Charles Fedele.

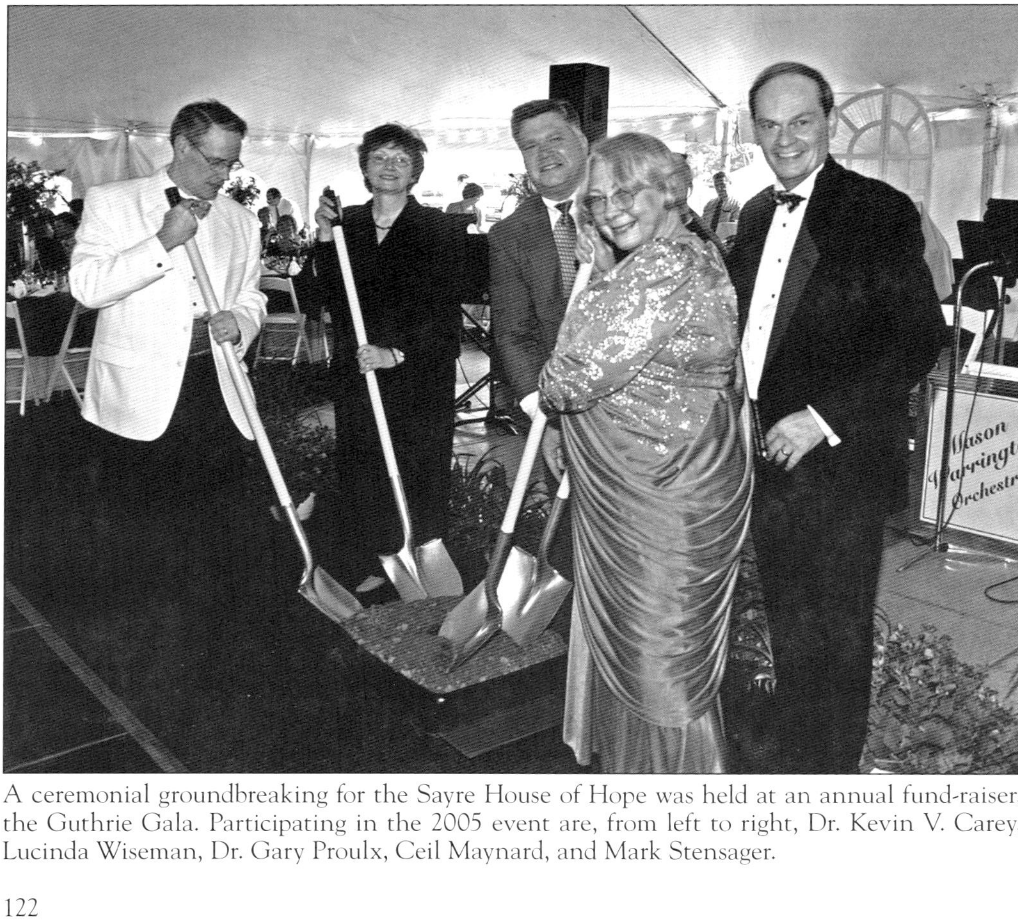

A ceremonial groundbreaking for the Sayre House of Hope was held at an annual fund-raiser, the Guthrie Gala. Participating in the 2005 event are, from left to right, Dr. Kevin V. Carey, Lucinda Wiseman, Dr. Gary Proulx, Ceil Maynard, and Mark Stensager.

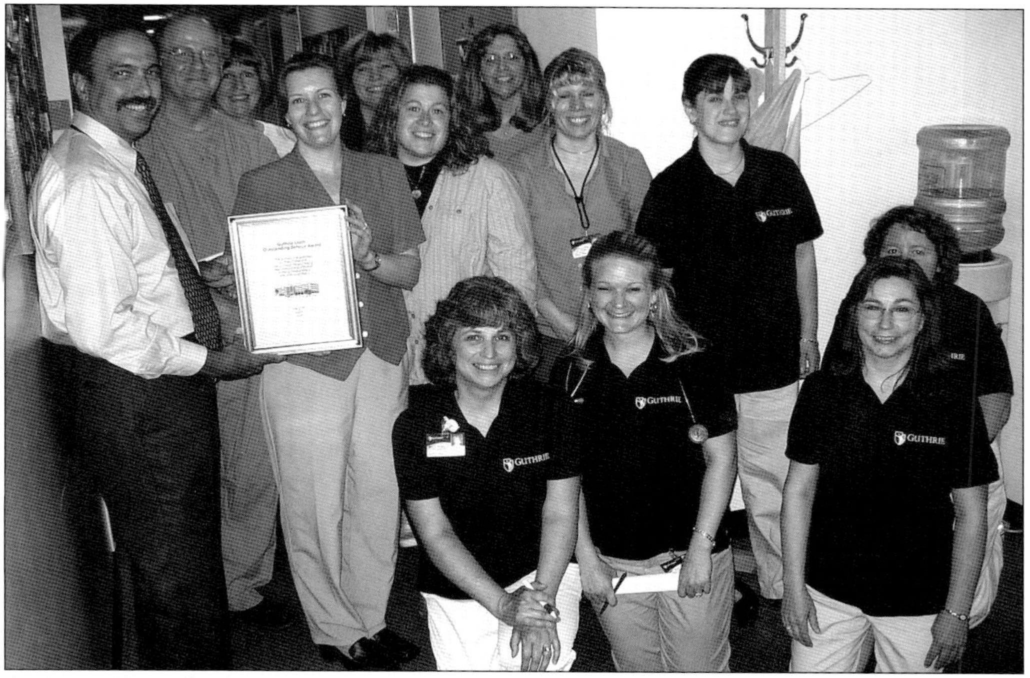

Guthrie Clinic leaders presented the 2005 Outstanding Service Awards to a number of departments and regional offices. The obstetrics and gynecology department in Sayre received a certificate of appreciation, presented by clinic president Dr. Joseph A. Scopelliti (far left).

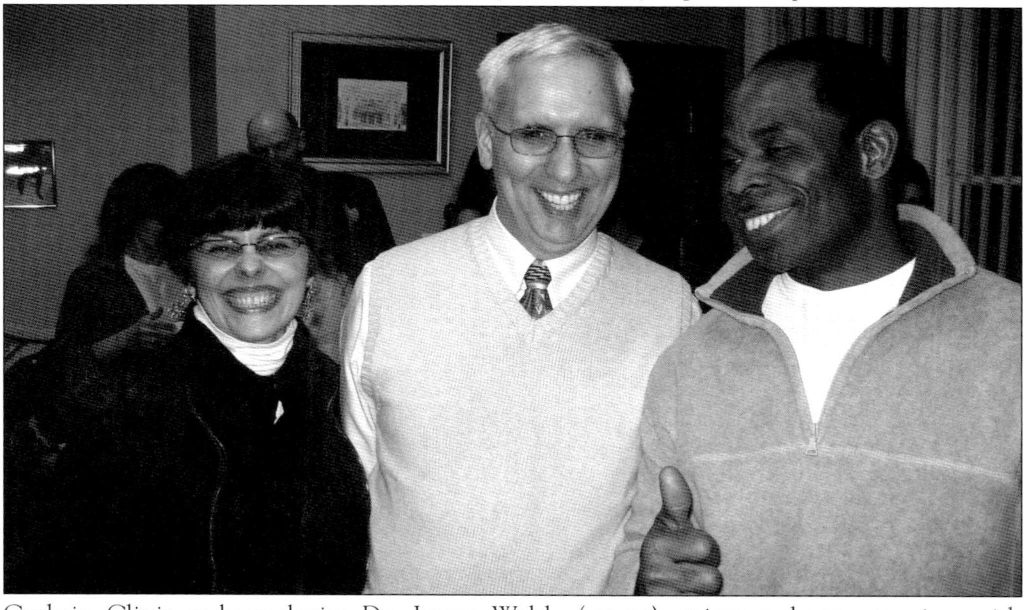

Guthrie Clinic pulmonologist Dr. James Walsh (center) enjoys a happy reunion with Vado Diomande (right) and Diomande's wife, Lisa. Diomande was a patient at the hospital for 35 days and received specialized care for treatment of inhalation anthrax. Because of the unusual diagnosis, the hospital and patient received media coverage throughout, and beyond, his hospitalization.

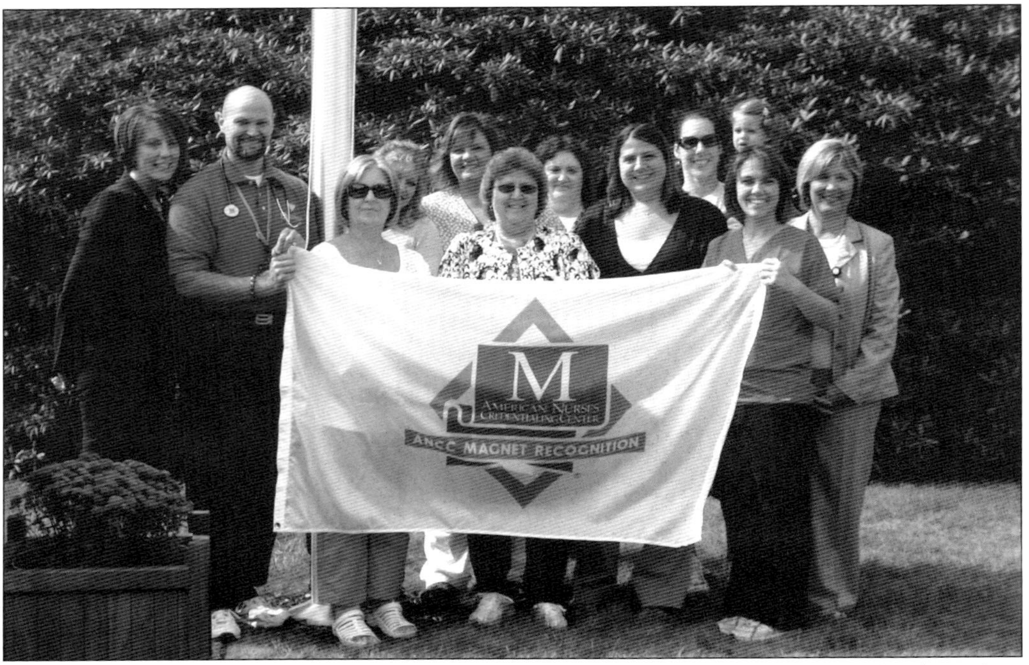

Robert Packer Hospital was designated a magnet hospital by the American Nurses Credentialing Center (ANCC) in 2008. For four years, the hospital's magnet team prepared for the ANCC assessment survey. Here members of the hospital magnet team proudly display the magnet flag.

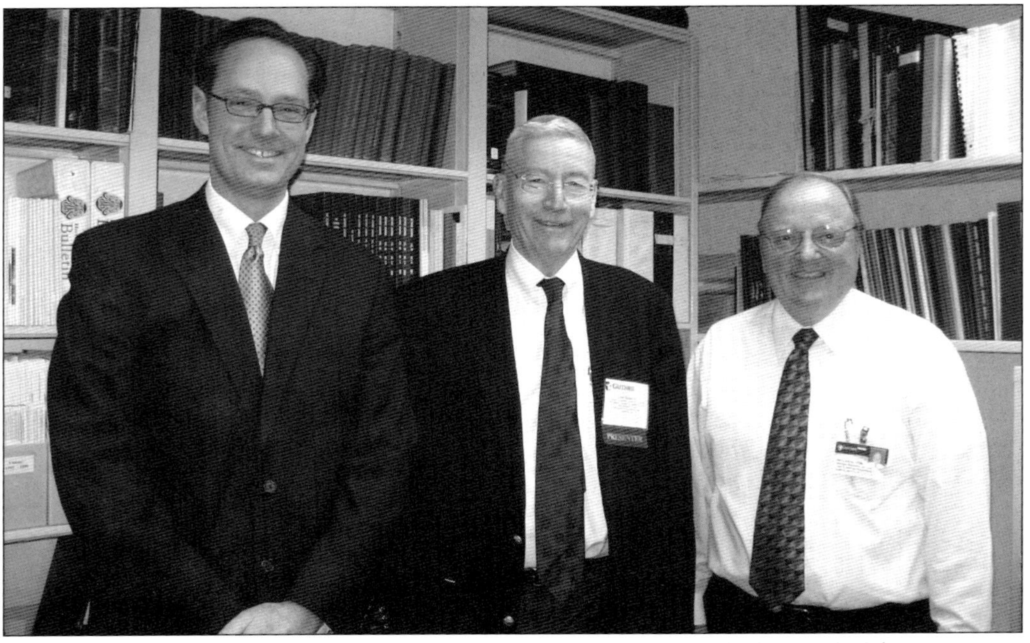

Dr. Clyde Barker, named the Donald Guthrie Professor of Surgery at the hospital of the University of Pennsylvania, came to Sayre in 2008 to present a lecture and receive a private tour of the Guthrie Archives. Shown here in the archives are, from left to right, Dr. Thomas VanderMeer, Dr. Barker, and Guthrie historian Henry Farley.

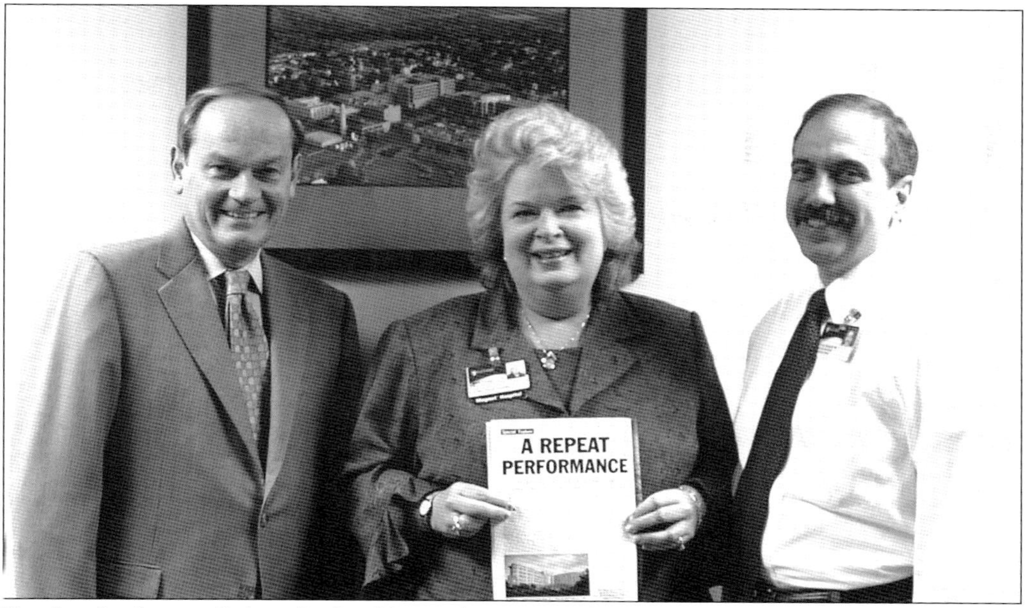

For the third time, Robert Packer Hospital was named to the list of 100 top hospitals. Shown here with the issue of *Modern Healthcare* that announced the 2008 winners are, from left to right, Guthrie Healthcare System chief executive officer Mark Stensager, Robert Packer Hospital chief operating officer Marie Droege, and Guthrie Clinic chief executive officer Dr. Joseph A. Scopelliti. In addition to winning this award three times, the hospital received the 100 top cardiovascular hospital award five times and the 100 top performance improvement award four times. The hospital also received the Everest Award in 2009, one of only 23 hospitals in the country to do so.

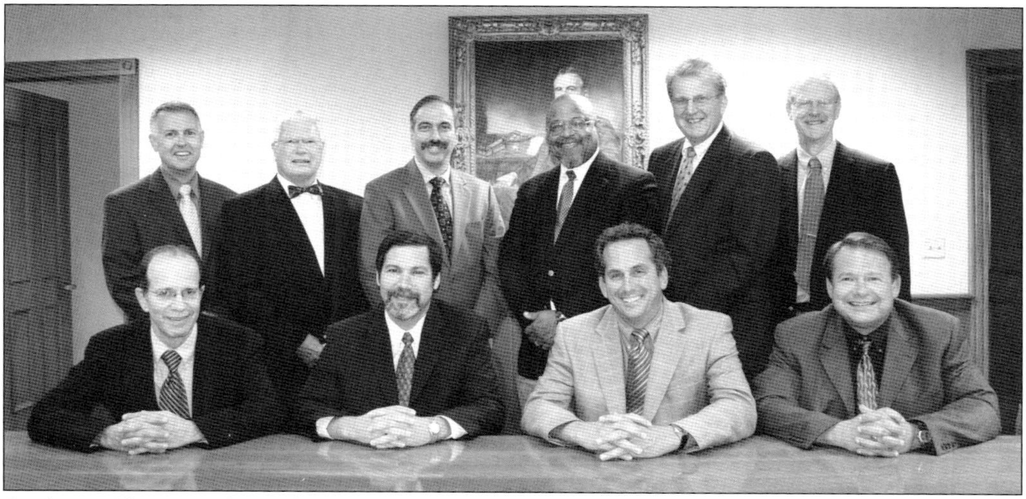

Guthrie Clinic and Guthrie Healthcare System continue to work closely together to provide access to the high-quality care patients expect and deserve. In this photograph is the 2009 Guthrie Clinic Board of Directors. From left to right are (first row) chairman Dr. Robert E. Cohen, secretary Dr. Daniel Sporn, Dr. David A. Talenti, and Dr. Mark Mauer; (second row) Dr. David Pfisterer, Dr. Edward L. Jones, president Dr. Joseph A. Scopelliti, treasurer Dr. Ferrol J. Lee, Dr. Douglas Trostle, and Dr. Thomas A. Yaeger.

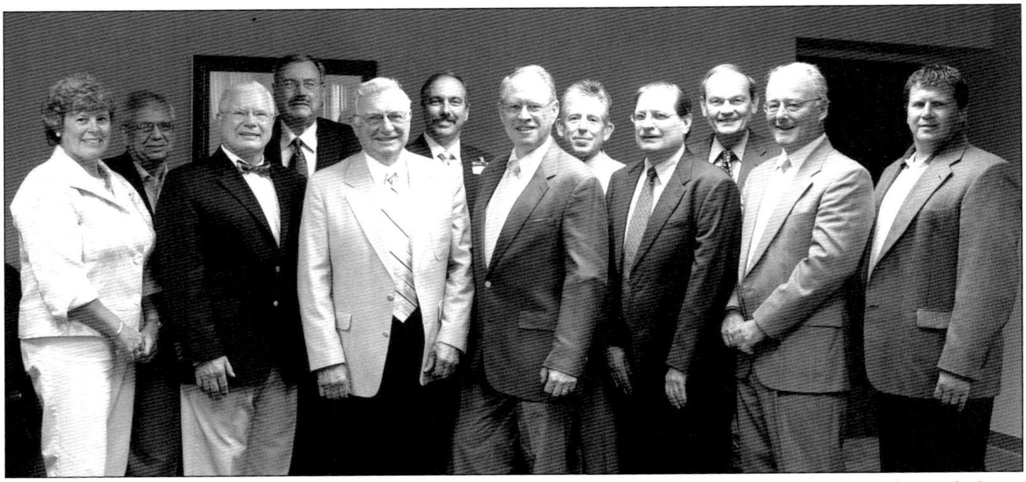

Members of the Guthrie Healthcare System Board of Directors in 2009 are, from left to right, Susan P. Storch, David E. Iocco, Dr. Edward L. Jones, chairman William H. Ransom III, David L. R. Gibbs, Dr. Joseph A Scopelliti, Dr. Kevin V. Carey, secretary-treasurer Richard W. Botnick, Kenneth R. Levitzky, Esq., president and chief executive officer Mark Stensager, vice chairman A. John Peck Jr., Esq., and Andrew Ripic.

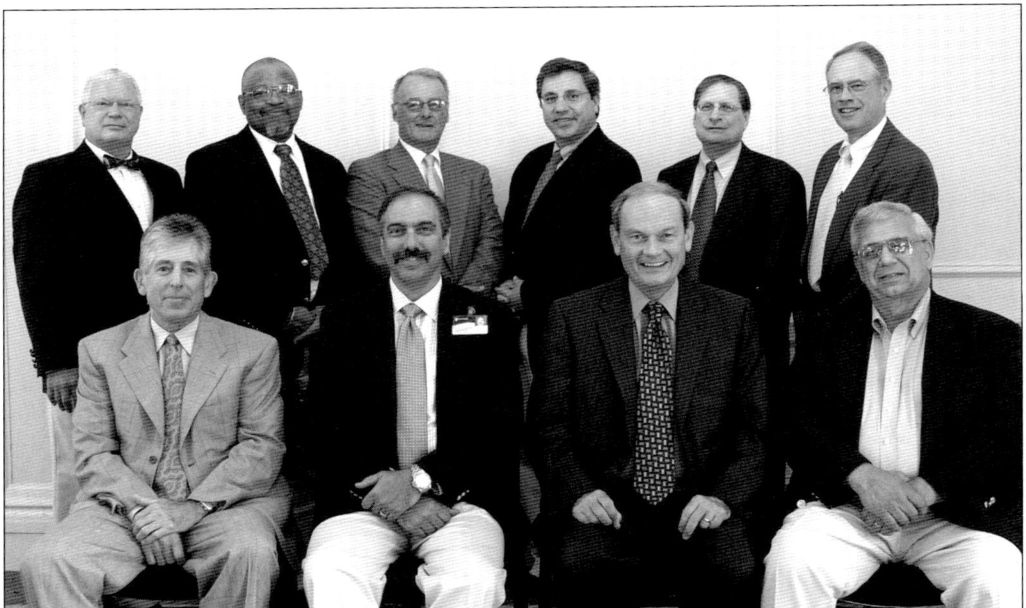

Pictured here are, from left to right, the Guthrie Health board members in 2009: (first row) chairman Richard W. Botnick, medical affairs co-chief executive officer Dr. Joseph A. Scopelliti, administrative affairs co-chief executive officer Mark Stensager, and David E. Iocco; (second row) treasurer Edward L. Jones, Dr. Ferrol J. Lee, A. John Peck Jr., Esq., Michael W. Donnelly, Kenneth R. Levizky, Esq., and Dr. Kevin V. Carey. Absent from the photograph are Dr. Kyra Bannister, Dr. Robert E. Cohen, vice chairman Dr. Terence Devine, and William H. Ransom III.

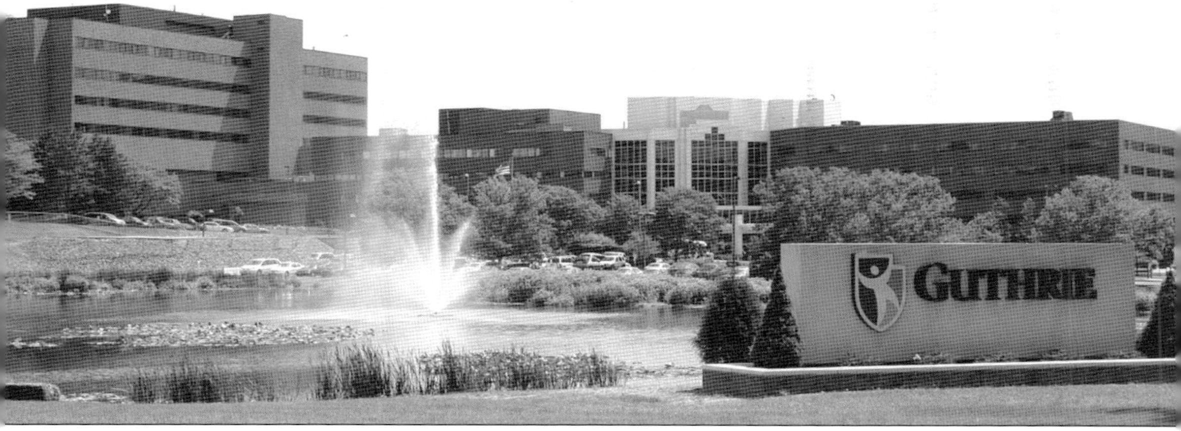

This photograph of Guthrie Health's Sayre campus was taken in 2009. Guthrie Health has grown significantly since Dr. Donald Guthrie's time. It now includes Robert Packer Hospital, a tertiary care hospital that serves as a regional level II trauma center; Corning Hospital, a community hospital; and Troy Community Hospital, a critical-access hospital. It also includes home care and hospice services, a skilled nursing facility, a durable medical equipment business, a research institute that offers numerous clinical trials, and physician offices in 23 communities.